Wilhelmine D. Schott

Health hints to women:

Important information for all

Wilhelmine D. Schott

Health hints to women:
Important information for all

ISBN/EAN: 9783337724184

Printed in Europe, USA, Canada, Australia, Japan

Cover: Foto ©ninafisch / pixelio.de

More available books at **www.hansebooks.com**

IINTS T

T INFORMATION

AND THE

CURE" EX

---

ve nor honor, wealth nor
ve the heart a cheerful h
health is lost. Be time
ealth all taste of pleasur

ELMINE D.

ner of the "Danis

WITH PORTRAIT.

REDERIC J. N

NEW YORK:

ARLES P. SOMERBY,

121 FOURTH AVENUE. ·

1883

CHARLES P. SOMERBY,
Printer and Electrotyper.

CONTENTS.

PART I.

PART II.

CONTENTS.

PART II.—Continued.

PART III.

PART III.—CONTINUED.

PART III.—Continued.

PART III.—CONTINUED.

———

PART IV.

PART V.

PART VI.

PART VI.—Continued.

PART VII.

PART VIII.

PREFACE.

THE design of the author of the following pages
has been to place within the reach of all women a
general outline of the laws of health, and of the conditions requisite thereto, and also such Health Hints as
shall enable them to guard against sickness, and to
understand just what to do for those who are sick.

Women, by virtue of their natural and social relations, have more to do with health and disease than *all
the doctors in the world*. They are our nurses in sickness ; they are the mothers and trainers of our children ; and, hence, they can do more to remove the diseases that afflict the human family than all the world
besides. How important, then, that they should be put
in possession of that knowledge that will qualify them
for the great duties devolving upon them.

The sufferings of women are of a peculiar and
aggravated nature. This is the result of her dependent
condition—of the peculiarities of her physical organization—of the special duties imposed on her as a

mother—and, above all, of her blind subserviency to the unreasonable restrictions and the health-destroying fashions and customs of society. And yet, while thus exposed in an eminent degree to disease, her dependence on man for aid and counsel, and her native modesty, subject her to peculiar disadvantages in seeking relief.

This little work is intended to obviate some of these difficulties ; and the author is sure that those for whom it is designed will gladly welcome a friend, that will forewarn them of the dangers at which she has hinted.

The prevalent amount of disease among women is *not* a sacred birthright, derived from the providential construction of things, but is *acquired*, and follows as the necessary consequence of the inharmonious action of the organism, imposed by the customs of society and the neglect of bodily culture.

It is thus that nervousness, dyspepsia, deformity of the spine and chest, the loss of the attractions which they should possess, and divers other afflictions which are so common, are fully accounted for.

The author has not designed to put out a system of medicine, or an *infallible* cure for everything, but to show that there is a real distinction between mechanical and vital disease, or those requiring mechanical and vital remedies, and that one *will not* answer the place of the other ; also, that the mechanical diseases, or causes of disease, are more common and extensive than is generally supposed.

Once the human system was looked upon as a mere moving mystery, without any rational comprehension of its structure and functions. Once the muscular system, by which all the movements of the body are propelled and made regular and efficient, was not at all understood. Once the circulation of the blood, by which the system is perpetuated and nourished, was not dreamed of; the best and wisest of the faculty supposed that blood flowed through the system, like water through a sponge. The function of assimilation, by which the food is turned to blood and flesh, was not conceived of; and many other matters like the above were chaotic, but now are perceived by every common understanding, and explained by the general action of matter on matter.

As the human economy is more perfectly understood, the more does it resemble a machine of great complexity and perfection; and, like a machine, is governed and propelled by the combined mechanical powers and philosophical laws that control all arrangements, and give order to their operations; thus reducing the science of life and disease to those great and tangible principles that are understood by every one; making the human economy appear sublime, as well as wonderful, and giving us rational cause to exclaim with the Psalmist, "For we are fearfully and wonderfully made."

For many years past, the author of this volume has been more and more impressed with the idea that the greatest portion of all the suffering, disease, deformity, and premature deaths which occur, are the direct result of either the violation of, or the want of compliance with, the laws of our being.

The physician, while he confines himself to the treatment and cure of disease and deformity, does nothing but plaster over the evils of humanity. He is at best but a simple scavenger—useful, it is granted, in a low degree—so long as he confines himself entirely to the removal of the effects, or symptoms and diseases, which are the result of causes still operative.

If he fails to point out to the community the causes of the ills which he is called upon to treat, and, if he does not by his own example strive to induce others to shun them, he is unworthy of that calling.

In the course of her practice, it has been the habit of the author to give her patients, from time to time, such hints and suggestions, with regard to the proper management of themselves and their children, as the occasion called for. These they have deemed of so much value as to wish to possess them in a convenient form for future use and reference. It is at their request, therefore, that the second edition of this book has been prepared for publication ; and at their hands it is sure to find a welcome. Her aim has been to furnish the reader with the greatest amount of useful information possible, in a small compass, and to give the why and the wherefore in language which all can understand.

The delicate subjects necessarily embraced in a work of this kind are treated with the utmost regard for decency and propriety, while all useless and non-essential revelations are excluded.

The class of persons who will best understand the meaning, as well as the method of the Danish Cure, consist of those who have been, or are, under her direction. Indeed, this is the class that loudly call for the work, and who have constantly spurred her on to its completion.

The importance of the Danish Cure in the correction of Spinal Deformities, Contractions, Paralysis, Dropsy, Soft Tumors, Kidney Diseases, Diseases of the Blood, Weakened Muscles, etc., and for preventing disease, can not be over-estimated.

It is conceived by the author, that the importance of animal electricity, employed as herein directed, as a curative resource, is second to that of no other heretofore brought before the public. It succeeds where medicines fail ; it strengthens more surely than any tonic ; it imparts electricity without the unpleasant

shock of the battery ; it soothes while it invigorates.
It may be considered as a means of enabling the
natural tendencies of the system toward health to act
more powerfully and effectually. It directs the cor-
poreal energies into just those channels in which they
are most needed, in order to perfect the balance of the
physiological processes. It enables the system to develop and maintain its forces in greater amount,
because it employs them naturally and without undue
waste.

While on the other hand the use of Drugs is too
frequently a dangerous experiment, and their employment, in mechanical chronic diseases, useless and
ridiculous.

HEALTH HINTS TO WOMEN.

——✳——

PART I.

CURE WITHOUT DRUGS.

POOR human nature! How fearfully does it deceive itself, when it flies to drugs to relieve every disease!

See that pale cheek, that eye that has lost its lustre, that care-worn countenance, that languid step, that flaccid muscle, with great weakness, and the indisposition to exertion, and you will behold a faithful picture of the evil results of drugging.

To discover truth in science, the most learned will admit, is very often difficult; but in no science is it more difficult than in that of medicine.

The time has arrived when the people of this country begin to read and think for themselves, to learn things and not words; to exercise their

2

judgment in matters which concern their welfare
and that of their families, instead of paying other
people to think for them.

Among the common people the wide distinction between Prevention and Cure has not
been generally recognized. They are apt to
think that all books relating to the laws of life
and health, must of course be treatises on diseases and cure by drugs.

They are, at least, often more eager to attain
reading matter in some contemptible quack doctor
book, which professes to teach them how to
doctor themselves, than they are apt to get books
to show how they destroy health and life, and
how to prevent diseases, broken constitutions
and premature death.

They regard *cure* infinitely more important
than *prevention.* As a general rule, they more
highly value a physician, who, instead of warning
them against the evils of violated law, will let
them go on unmolested till they have ruined
themselves, and then will be on hand to drug
them thoroughly, even unto death, than they

will that person who has the moral courage in the cause of humanity, who peril their reputation to prevent them from encountering needless suffering, and an early grave.

They want their false appetites and ruinous indulgences to be let alone ; and when health is gone, as a consequence, they want a doctor, or doctor's book, to prescribe drugs which promise to restore health in spite of their continuing the indulgence which caused it. Or, if they set aside the cause for a short space, they want to be so thoroughly drugged that Nature may never dare to make such another outcry, so that they may turn to their sins with hopeful impunity.

At all events, they consider *health* a secondary matter—a matter of small importance until it is ruined, and then mourn over their pains and sufferings, when it is too late to make amends.

They practically consider the old proverb to be obsolete : " An ounce of prevention is worth more than a pound of cure." They persist in going on with their unnatural indulgences, undermining their physical vitality, until Nature, unable to bear abuse any longer, gives signs of woe. Then they resort, perhaps, to cures which only cure by death.

The first step toward the cure of diseases is effected by removing causes. Unless the original cause of any given disease be removed, there is no successful way of obtaining a permanent cure; and by the removal of the original cause, perhaps in more than nine cases out of ten, Nature will remove the difficulty without the aid of any kind of medicine.

It is the most consummate quackery to prescribe medicine to cure disease, while the cause that produced it is not abandoned. If a liver complaint, or kidney complaint, or any other glandular derangement shall occur, which has been produced by coffee, tea, or any other narcotic or stimulant, it is an outrage on all common sense, as well as science, to prescribe remedies while indulgence in these false luxuries is continued.

They must be abandoned, or health given up; and it is folly to inquire which should be relinquished. If proved to be hurtful they should be rejected.

Here comes a lady with prostrated nervous system, and from this arises a diversity of complaints ; dyspepsia in its various forms and its hundred attendant sufferings; sick headaches and nervous headaches, with their periodical visits, goneness at the stomach and palpitation of the heart ;—all of these, and many more, are caused by an over use of stimulating drink and hurtful food.

If the liver is the point to which her illegal living has directed its force, and her immediate sufferings arise from a torpid condition of that gland, accompanied with its usual attendant, a sluggish condition of the bowels, she runs after some nostrum in the form of anti-bilious pills, or other quackery.

She takes her pills, which force a temporary action that is generally followed by greater prostration of nervous force, giving the liver greater torpidity, and still continues her former mode of diet. This is like a woman holding her hand in

the fire till the skin is removed, calling on the
doctor for a salve, while she is still holding her
hand in the flame.   If she wants the burned skin
to be removed and a new one to take its place,
she must remove her hand from the fire; she
must first put away the original cause.   When
she does this, Nature will want little help to bring
things again to their right bearings.

Nature requires no help from medical agents,
and will perform her work of cure better and
more thoroughly without than with them.   Nature always goes for health; and so zealous is she
in her undertakings, and so certain of the best
possible issue, that we may rest assured that on
her part no pains will be spared, and on our part
no risk is run.

As before remarked, probably in nine cases
out of ten of all the diseases in the world, especially those of chronic form, where the primary
cause is removed, medicines do more harm than
good, for all medical agents are unnatural to the
laws of healthy life.

The philosophy of allopathic cure consists in

creating an unnatural condition of the animal economy, in opposition to the existing one. A morbid condition now exists; another morbid condition is instituted in order to overcome and expel it, and if the medicine succeed in removing it, still Nature must remove the unnatural condition produced by the medicine; and if Nature alone can remove any existing disease by having its cause removed, she will come out better in the end, than she will if two morbid conditions, instead of one, are thrown in her way.

My department of the medical profession has always been proficient in attention to the laws which govern health. The study of Pathology or the laws which govern diseased life, do not, as a general rule, direct sufficient attention to the laws which govern healthy life.

If those who are suffering ill health will read and inform themselves on the natural laws of healthy life, and cease violating them altogether, Nature will generally perform a cure. Seeking for remedies short of this is the worst of folly. It is spending time and money to no purpose,

and wasting the vital energies by medicines
which, when they cannot effect good, are only
increasing disease and hastening premature death.
If, instead of resorting to drug shops and quack
doctor books, women would see that all violations of natural law were put away, so that no
embarrassment should oppress Nature, they would
not only save themselves from a vast waste of
money, but from many a ruined constitution and
loss of life, which silver and gold cannot replace.

Oh, what consummate fools some people are!
If we recommend them a book on the laws of
health, they call it quackery, or a humbug. Or, if
we tell them at the bedside that they really need
no drugs, they will think us ignoramuses, and
probably send for some doctor so destitute of
skill or honesty, that he will abundantly gratify
them with medicines. The efforts of an honest
person they cannot appreciate ; but the man who
will furnish them with a doctor book, promising
to show them how to cure themselves with medicine—the man who will really humbug for money
—they will regard as a benefactor to the race.

The doctor who makes a display of powders and drops, which are only preparing them to drop into the ground, is at once reckoned one of the most skillful doctors of the age.

The man who will seek a reputation at the peril of the community, has not that degree of honesty which could prepare him for a station of such responsibility. He is obtaining money under false pretences, and even bartering the life that has been entrusted to his hands for paltry gain. Nay, he is worse than a highway robber and murderer. He meets you, not in a bold frank attitude of his real character, as does the highwayman, letting you understand at once your danger and need of preparation for defence, but comes to you in the meanest hypocrisy, pretending to be devoted to the cause of humanity and the relief of human suffering, while he is willing to let you go on in your course of self-destruction, and then, instead of seeking to show you wherein you have departed from Nature's path, and turn you back into it again, will deal out needless drugs, for money and a reputation, which push you into the grave.

Considering the ignorance of too many of the American people, and their fondness for drugs— the increased indifference to the laws of health because there are plenty of doctors and medicine on hand—it is pretty safe to conclude, that the standard of health and longevity would be far above its present position, if medicines had never been known in the land, and not a physician had ever set foot upon its soil.

The existence of medicines and physicians will probably continue to do more harm than good, until the friends of humanity will take more interest in diffusing among the people a knowledge of the laws of the human system which relate to practical life, and a thorough knowledge of anatomy. Then, and not till then, will doctors and medicines become, on the whole, blessings to the community.

PHILOSOPHY OF MEDICINE DENIED.

The system of the healing art which I advocate and practice, not only repudiates all the remedies of the mineral drug order, but denies the philosophy on which their employment is predicated. It charges their practice with being *destructive*, and their theory with being *false*. It ignores the fundamental premises of all drug-medical systems, and declares the truth to be the exact contrary of what they teach.

To illustrate : it is taught in all their books and schools, that Nature has provided remedies for diseases in the things *outside of the domain of organic life.* The truth is exactly the contrary. Nature has provided *penalties*, and among them sickness, as the consequences of disobedience to organic law ; but she has not provided *remedies to do away the penalties.*

It is also taught in all their schools and books that disease is an entity — a thing foreign to the living organism, and an enemy to the life-principle. The truth is exactly the contrary. Disease is the *life-principle itself at war with an enemy.* It is the defender and protector of the living organism ; it is a process of purification ; it is an effort to remove foreign and offensive materials from the system, and to repair the damages the vital machinery has sustained.

Disease, therefore, is not a foe to be subdued or killed, but a friendly office, to be directed and regulated, and every attempt to subdue disease with drug poisons is nothing more nor less than a war on the human constitution.

Physicians occasionally arise who have the magnanimity to admit that they can calculate with no certainty on their medicines, these utterly failing under the most favorable combination of symptoms to exhibit those effects, for the production of which it is supposed they are specifically adapted.

Thus calomel, opium, quinine, lobelia, belladonna, aconite, toxicodendron, arsenic, iodine, podophyllin, and the other poisons whose name is legion, and in whose tails there are a thousand stings, are daily given, and specified effects are looked for and calculated upon, but exactly opposite effects are produced.

Am I not right? If not, how then is opium given to induce sleep, and the patient made all the more wakeful for it? Is it not a common fact that calomel, when administered with a view to excite the liver to increased action, produces, as a result, greater inactivity of that organ? Do not physicians daily give cathartics to relieve costiveness, and thereby make it a permanent condition of the bowels? Do they not give cantharides to cure dropsy, and then have to commence the process of tapping, and keep it up till the patient dies?

Do they not give iodine to reduce enlarged lymphatics, and have suppuration of the glands follow its administration? Do they, or do they not get results such as the books tell about, in half the cases they treat? I do not ask if their patients live through the attacks of their diseases and the administrative attendance of their physicians. That is not just now the question; but do these medicine givers with their so-called specifics get specific effects?

The treatment of diseases with drugs ever was, now is, and always must be, uncertain and dangerous experimentation. It never was and never can be reduced to reliable practical rules. An art is the application of the principles of a science to specific results; and a science is an arrangement of ascertained principles in their normal order and relations. These principles constitute the premises of the system, which is made up of the science and the art. But in medicine, according to the philosophy of all the drug schools, every one of its fundamental premises is false; hence its science is false, and its practice must be false also.

On the contrary, the Danish Cure, or the treatment of diseases by manipulation, is founded on the demonstrable laws of physiology, and reducible to fixed and invariable rules of practice, and it affords the data for a true Medical Science and a successful Healing Art.

Wherever and by whomsoever this system is understood, it is adopted. Just so fast as people become thoroughly acquainted with it, they abandon all the systems of drug-medication.

Thenceforth they have very little need of the physician, and never patronize the quack. They will not be killed by *regular*, nor imposed upon by *irregular*, physicians.

All that I have said, shall say, or can say

against drug-medication, and in favor of the Danish Cure, is more than confirmed by the standard authors and living teachers of the drug-system. Here let me introduce to my readers some of the most eminent professors of Medical Colleges in these United States.

Said the venerable Professor Alexander H. Stephens, M. D., of the New York College of Physicians and Surgeons, in a recent lecture to the medical class : "The older physicians grow, the more skeptical they become of the virtues of medicine, and the more they are disposed to trust to the powers of Nature." Again : "Notwith-standing all our boasted improvement, patients suffer as much as they did forty years ago." And again : "The reason medicine has advanced so slowly, is because physicians have studied the writings of their predecessors, instead of Nature."

The venerable Professor Jos. M. Smith, M. D., of the same school, testifies : "All medicines which enter the circulation, *poison the blood* in the same manner as do the poisons that pro-duce disease." Again : "Drugs do not cure disease; disease is always cured by vis medicatrix naturæ."

Says Professor Alonzo Clark, M.D., of the same school: " In their zeal to do good, physicians have done much harm. They have *hurried many to the grave* who would have recovered if left to Nature. All of our curative agents are poisons, and, as a consequence, *every dose diminishes the patient's vitality.*"

Says Professor J. W. Carson, M.D., of the New York Medical College: " It is easy to destroy the life of an infant. You will find that a slight scratch of the pen, which indicates a little too much remedy, *will snuff out the infant's life;* and when you next visit your patient, you will find that the child which you left cheerful a few hours previously, is *stiff and cold.* Beware, then, how you use your remedies." Again: " We do not know whether our patients recover because we give medicine, or because Nature cures them. Perhaps *bread pills* would cure as many as medicine."

Says Professor E. S. Carr, M.D., of the New

York University Medical School : "All drugs
are more or less adulterated, and as not more
than one physician in a hundred has sufficient
knowledge in chemistry to detect impurities, the
physician seldom knows just how much of a
remedy he is prescribing." Again, " Mercury,
when administered in any form, is taken into the
circulation, and carried to every tissue of the
body. The effects of mercury are not for a day
or a year, *but for all time.* It often lodges in
the bones, occasionally causing pain *years after
it is administered.* I have often detected metallic
mercury in the bones of patients who had been
treated with this *subtle poisonous agent.*"

Says Professor B. F. Barker, M.D., of the
same school : " The drugs which are administered
for the cure of scarlet fever and measles, *kill far
more than those diseases do.* I have recently
given *no medicine* in their treatment, and have
had excellent success." Again : " I am inclined
to think that mercury, in any form, given to
patients does *far more harm than good.*" And
again ; " Instead of investigating for themselves,

3

medical authors have *copied the errors* of their predecessors, and have thus retarded the progress of medical science and perpetuated error."

Says Professor Parker : " As we place more confidence in Nature and less in preparations of the apothecary, *mortality diminishes.*" Again : " Hygiene is of *far more value* in the treatment of diseases than drugs. I have cured granulations of the eyes, in chronic conjunctivitis, by Hygienic treatment, after all kinds of drug-applications had failed."

Says Professor Clark : " A hundred different and unsuccessful plans have been tried for the cure of cholera. I think I shall leave my patients hereafter nearly entirely to Nature, as I have seen patients abandoned to die and left to Nature recover, while patients who were treated died."

Says Benjamin Rush, M.D., Professor of the Medical College in Philadelphia : " I am incessantly led to make an apology for the instability of the theories and practice of physic. Those physicians generally become the most eminent who have most thoroughly emancipated themselves from the tyranny of the schools of medicine. Dissections daily convince us of our *ignorance of disease*, and cause us to blush at our prescriptions. What *mischiefs* have we not done under the belief of *false facts* and *false theories?* We have assisted in *multiplying diseases;* we have done more: we have *increased their fatality."*

Says Dr. Ramage, Fellow of the Royal College, London: " It cannot be denied that the present system of medicine is a *burning shame* to its professors, if indeed a series of vague and uncertain incongruities deserves to be called by that name. How rarely do our medicines do good! How often do they make our patients *really worse!* I fearlessly assert that in most cases the sufferer would be *safer without a doctor* than with one. I have seen enough of the *malpractice* of my professional brethren to warrant the strong language I employ."

Look at this also:

" Some patients get well with the aid of medicine ; more without it ; and still more *in spite of it."*—Sir John Forbes, M. D., *Physician* to Queen Victoria.

"Thousands are annually *slaughtered* in the quiet sick-room. Governments should at once either banish medical men, and proscribe their *blundering art*, or they should adopt some better means to protect the lives of the people than at present prevail, when they look far less after the practice of this *dangerous profession*, and the murders committed in it, than after the lowest trades."—Dr. Frank, an eminent European Author and Practitioner.

" I may observe, that of the whole number of fatal cases in infancy, a great proportion occur from the inappropriate or undue application of *exhausting remedies*."—Dr. Marshall Hall, the distinguished English Physiologist.

" Our actual information or knowledge of disease does not increase in proportion to our experimental practice. Every dose of medicine given is a *blind experiment upon the vitality* of the patient."—Dr. Bostock, author of the " History of Medicine."

These extracts, which might very easily be extended so as to fill a large volume, shall conclude with the following confession and declaration, deliberately adopted and recorded by the members of the National Medical Convention, representing the *elite* of the profession of the United States, held in St. Louis, Mo., a few years ago :

" It is wholly incontestable that there exists a widespread dissatisfaction with what is called the regular, or old allopathic system of medical practice. Multitudes of people in this country and in Europe express an utter want of confidence in physicians and their physic. The cause is evident : *erroneous theory*, and springing from it, *injurious* —often, very often—FATAL PRACTICE ! Nothing will now subserve the absolute requisitions of an intelligent community but medical treatment grounded upon *right reason*, in harmony with, and avouched by the *unerring laws of nature* and of the vital organism, and authenticated and confirmed by successful results."

Such being the deliberate assertions, declarations, and confessions of those who advocate, teach, and practice the drug system, would it not be well, my reader, to avoid this fatal treatment with dangerous drugs, and turn your attention to a milder and more effectual treatment—one based strictly on the fundamental principles of nature?

PART II.

FOOD.

"In what thou eat'st and drinkest seek from thence
Due nourishment, not gluttonous delight ;
So thou may'st live till, like ripe fruit, thou drop
Into thy mother's lap, or be with ease
Gather'd, not harshly pluck'd, for death mature."

THE tissues of our bodies are constantly wearing out. We cannot perform a single act, or even think, without wearing out some portion of the tissues, and these require to be constantly replenished ; otherwise, the whole body would soon be used up.

It is this wearing-out process that creates a demand for food, and, as with all other things, so with the body ; its nature, form, properties, and other qualities, depend largely on the nature and properties of the material from which it is constructed.

In order that our bodies may be properly maintained, it is necessary that our food should be just adapted to the wants of our system.

The food we eat should contain all the elements required to build up the body, otherwise some parts, or the whole of the system, will be improperly sustained.

If our food is mingled with, or contains elements that are not usable in the system, the organs of depuration have additional work to do in removing these unusable elements from the system, and this extra work will soon wear them out.

Pain is a symptom, not a disease. Rightly understood, it is a friend ; it comes to tell us, in tones neither to be mistaken nor ignored, that we have violated the laws of health and must suffer the consequences. It bids us to examine ourselves in respect to food, exercise, clothing, work and play, and see wherein we have offended and need to repent and amend.

Too much is eaten, or too little, or is eaten too hurriedly, or at the wrong time, or of the wrong kinds. Yet it is impossible to mark out any single regimen that will suit all classes, ages, occupations, habits and conditions of health.

The one thing necessary for a woman to understand, is that certain kinds of food furnish certain elements to her body, indispensable to its growth and health—some in a greater, some in a less degree—and should not therefore be accepted or rejected ignorantly, indifferently, or capriciously, but carefully selected with a view to their power of repairing bodily waste, and accelerating or retarding the bodily functions.

Afterward she must study and experiment for herself, to ascertain what kinds and proportions of farinaceous, vegetable, and animal food are best suited to her peculiar constitution and circumstances. No doubt she will make some mistakes at first, but she will do much better than if she eats blindly whatever comes to hand, without other aim than present gratification.

Yet care should be taken not to err on the side of abstemiousness. Nearly *all* varieties of food are useful in their proper place and proportion.

Regularity should be observed in the time of eating, for the digestive organs become weary by long-continued labor, and require rest.   In order that they may obtain this rest, it is necessary that the food should be taken at stated times, and never until the previous meal has been digested, and the stomach has had sufficient time to rest.

The quantity of food taken at a meal has also an important influence upon the health.

If food is taken in too great quantities, or too frequently, it cannot be properly digested, consequently the health and strength of the body will not be properly maintained, and a great amount of the vital force will be expended in expelling this same improperly digested food.   For food which has not been properly digested is not usable, and is regarded by the system as a poison. The .American people, as a general rule, eat altogether too frequently to be healthy.   After a child is five or six years of age it should not be allowed to eat more than three times in the twenty-four hours, unless it is sick and able to take only a very little nutriment at a time.   It is this pernicious habit of eating between meals that ruins the stomach, and thus undermines the constitution of children.

They do not eat because they are hungry ; for such children know nothing of real hunger. They have a morbid appetite, an unnatural craving, but this is not hunger.

Infants under one year of age should take food four or five times in the twenty-four hours at regular intervals, after they are one year old, three meals a day will be far better than more in the majority of cases, but of this the mother or nurse must be the judge in each case.

Women who have always been in the habit of eating three meals a day, or of eating late suppers, usually rise in the morning with but little appetite for breakfast. This is because they fall asleep with undigested food in their stomachs, and a part of the organs had to remain awake to digest this food, consequently, the sleep was not as refreshing as it would have been, had all of the organs rested and slept together, and especially is this true of the stomach.

The stomach is in direct connection with the brain by means of the pneumogastric nerve ; therefore, when the stomach is actively at work, the brain must of necessity be more or less disturbed.

It is for this reason that hearty late suppers should never be indulged in. Those who have properly tried the two-meal system invariably find that they are much better able to endure severe protracted labor, either mental or physical, than they were when in the habit of eating three times a day, and, in addition, they find that their sleep is much more refreshing, they are not troubled with sour stomach, heartburn, eructations, etc., unless they over-eat, which is sometimes the case with those who eat but twice a day.

THE KIND OF FOOD.

Each species of animal is just adapted to subsist on certain kinds of food. Some species will thrive and maintain themselves in good condition on certain kinds of food, upon which other animals would starve.

Various as are the species belonging to the animal kingdom, they all derive their food either directly, or indirectly, from the vegetable kingdom. It is true that some classes of animals subsist wholly upon animal flesh, and that other classes make flesh a large portion of their aliment, yet the animals that are thus eaten derive their nourishment directly from the vegetable kingdom, so that all the nourishment taken by even the flesh-eating animals is derived indirectly from the vegetable kingdom.

The reason why one animal can subsist upon food upon which another would starve, is that the digestive apparatus of each species of animal is just adapted to digest certain special kinds of food, and no other kind of food can be so readily converted into blood as can that to which the digestive organs are adapted.

An examination of the organs of the various species of animals, and of their habits when in a state of nature, with no artificial habits, will show us why one animal can subsist on small twigs and boughs of bushes or trees, while another uses straw or hay, and yet another subsists wholly upon grain, while a fourth uses no other food than fruit.

There is no doubt but that man can subsist for a time, at least, upon very many kinds of vegetable substances, and also upon most kinds of flesh.

Flesh meat is not as good food, nor as healthy as vegetable substances. It contains no nutrient property that can not be obtained from vegetable substances, since the animal from which the flesh is obtained derived its nourishment from the vegetable kingdom.

All flesh, even while the animal is still in life and health contains more or less broken-down tissue in a state of decomposition. After the animal has been slaughtered, decomposition speedily becomes much more extensive and rapidly progresses to putrefaction. In fact, freshly slaughtered flesh is not considered by epicures as being as palatable as that which has been slaughtered a few days. It is not sweet, juicy, or tender as it is after the process of decomposition has commenced.

These three properties are all due to its

partial decomposition, hence as a rule, flesh meat should be well cooked, the cooking process destroys the injurious effect which is caused by partial decomposition.

Many physicians recommend flesh meat to be eaten when rare, this is beneficial only to the extent of mastication, as rare meat is generally masticated more thoroughly than tender, well cooked meat. My experience has been that rare meat has a very decided tendency to create tape and pin-worms. In well-cooked meat this objective tendency is removed.

THE BEST FOOD.

Beef is the best animal food, and should be most frequently used, it is easily digested and furnishes the body with many necessary properties requisite to its maintenance.

I have often seen a convalescent much troubled by a bowl of delicate broth, when a half dozen mouthfuls of beef-steak containing twice the quantity of nourishment, could be readily assimilated by the stomach.

In the first case the organ was distended, embarrassed, the gastric juice diluted, in the other, this fluid was in its full strength, and the organ would give its undivided powers to the digestion of the small mass within it.

Ladies who exercise much should eat meat at least once a day. To those who exercise very little a vegetable diet would probably be more beneficial.

Mutton appears to be a meat more easily digested than beef. This is not appreciated by a healthy person because the digestive power is in excess of what is required for the easy digestion of either, when a proper amount only is consumed.

In the dyspeptic, however, where a nice balance may exist between the digestive power possessed and that required, the usual experience is that mutton taxes the stomach less than beef, with invalids or persons of weak digestion, mutton will often be found more beneficial, than any other kind of meat.

Veal and lamb although more tender, are

more resistant to the digestive organs. They appear also to possess less . strength-giving properties.

It need scarcely be said that there is a deeply rooted belief that for sustaining the powers under great exertion these meats are not to be compared to beef and mutton. They are meats that it is desirable to avoid, generally speaking, in cases of dyspepsia.

Pork is rich and trying to the stomach on account of the large quantity of fat it contains. Doctors as a rule condemn pork because they say it is *indigestible* (?) A substance may be very nutritive, and yet very difficult of digestion, and on the other hand it may be easy of digestion, and yet may afford but little nourishment. The nutritiveness of an article of food, is measured by the amount of material it may furnish for building up the body.

The digestibility of food, is determined by the facility with which it is dissolved and changed by the stomach, etc. If our food be too dense and close in its texture the process of digestion

4

will be retarded. Now I maintain, that because
of the looseness of the texture of pork it is *not*
indigestible, but is *easily* digested, and will be
found very beneficial to women who are suffering
from weak lungs, or any pulmonary ailment.

Of course, fatty substances, are always more
in order in cold weather than in warm, as they
yield a large amount of carbon, and consequently
of heat to the body.

Venison partakes more of the character of
game than of butcher's meat. Its flesh is lean,
dark-colored, and savory. It constitutes one of
the most digestible of meats, and would be, therefore, well suited for the dyspeptic and convalescent were it not for its rich and savory character.

Next to mammals, or animals that suckle their
young, birds are of the most importance to us in
the selection of healthy food.

As far as it is known, there is no bird, and no
part of any bird, nor any bird's egg, which may
not be safely used as food. It must be stated,
however, that some birds render themselves
poisonous by the food which they eat.

The pheasant, for instance, which feeds on poisonous buds, is deemed poisonous during winter and spring. The flesh of birds differ from that of mammals in never being marbled or having fat mixed with the muscular fibres.

The flesh of game contains a smaller amount of fat than that of poultry, but it possesses more strengthening properties, and is also tender and easy of digestion. It possesses a marked and delicate flavor which increases by keeping.

The flavor of the partridge and quail is exceedingly delicate, and so also is that of the snipe and woodcock, but these latter birds are richer. From the qualities possessed by it, game is tempting to the invalid. Its easy digestibility, renders it further well suited to a weak stomach.

The wild turkey and goose are far more preferable, as an article of food, than the domesticated bipeds which we find so frequently upon our tables.

It is a well-known fact that game contributes more largely to our supply of blood than domesticated animals of the same species.

Chicken possesses no strength but nourishment. The white meat of a chicken possesses very little nourishment and is not readily digested. It should therefore be avoided where weakness of the stomach exists.

Fish is an important article of food. A very large number of different kinds — both freshwater and salt are consumed, giving great variety to this kind of food.

The amount that must exist in the vast waters of the ocean, may also be regarded as rendering the supply inexhaustible. As an article of nourishment, fish does not possess the satisfying and stimulating properties that belong to the flesh of quadrupeds and birds.

Still, as a less stimulating article of food than meat, fish possess valuable properties in a therapeutic point of view, and is constantly being advantageously employed when the powers are too weak for stronger kinds of animal food to be borne.

Fish also renders valuable assistance to the kidneys, in the performance of their duty.

Dr. Davy says, " If we give our attention to classed people — classed as to the quality of food they principally subsist on — we shall find that the class who subsist principally on fish, are especially strong, healthy, and prolific. In no other class than in that of fishers do we see larger families, handsomer women, or more robust and active men."

Fish contain a great deal of electricity, and as the stomach is directly connected with the brain, the electricity passes thence and the effect produced is very beneficial. This is the reason fish is commonly called " brain food."

In Denmark women are given boiled fish, three days after confinement, in preference to any other article of food.

MILK.

Milk is an article intended by nature as the sole food for the young of a certain class of animals, it necessarily contains all the elements that are required for the growth and maintenance of the body.

Good milk is a very white or a faintly buff-tinted liquid, which is entirely free from any viscidity, and undergoes no change on being heated. It has a sweet taste and a slightly perceptible agreeable odor.

The ingredients of milk consist of

Nitrogenous matter,

Fatty matter,

Sugar of milk,

Mineral matter and water.

It will be seen from this brief notice of the composition of milk, that it is a highly compound nourishment.

In this we find an illustration of the truth, that no single element of food will support life, for in milk is provided water to distend the stomach, dilute, wash out, nourish, etc., butter and oil for heat, and lime for making the bones solid and for other purposes.

Albumen, one of the nutritive elements of milk, rises to the surface in the form of a thin scum on boiling, this may be skimmed off, and the milk may thus be made more digestible for weak stomachs, but at the same time it will be less nourishing. Therefore milk should not be boiled and skimmed where a very nourishing diet is required. Milk without any preparation is very digestible and easily converted into our bodies, and it does not cause that heat, and excitement, that generally arise from the use of other kinds of animal food.

Being composed largely of water, it is readily absorbed by the stomach, and as the solid portions only are digested, a large quantity of milk really imposes less labor on the stomach than an equal quantity of any other food.

Very soon after milk is swallowed it is curdled by the action of the stomach, and as the act of vomiting is very easy in children, any excess of curd, that might oppress the stomach, is readily thrown off.

Milk varies somewhat in different animals, that of the goat approaching human milk more nearly than the milk of any other animal.

Butter and cheese though they are generally easily managed by the stomach, as they exist in combination with milk, are yet rather hard of digestion when in a separate state.

Old cheese is highly indigestible except when eaten with other indigestible food, it then acts as an assistant to digestion. Butter is not so objectionable, but its oily nature makes it a bad thing for weak stomachs.

Before dismissing the subject of milk, it may be well to add that the vomiting of curd, so common in children, is no evidence of disease, but rather evidence of health ; curdling of the milk being the natural effect of the gastric juice. But while the vomiting of curd is no symptom of actual disease, it is an evidence of injurious overloading of the stomach, which is quite a common error, and did not Nature relieve herself by vomiting, many more children would be sacrificed than there are. Many women say that milk does not agree with them ; that it causes constipation, etc. *Boiled milk only* causes constipation. By adding a little lime that cause will be removed. It is well known that fresh milk is very digestible and quite frequently causes diarrhœa.

If the liver is active and in a healthy condition, a woman can eat any kind of food. In nine cases out of ten where the physicians say the stomach is out of order, because it refuses certain kinds of food, the liver will be found to be the seat of trouble.

The liver is the regulator of our system, if that be wrong, all is wrong. Can we expect our digestion to be good when the liver is inactive and in an unhealthy condition? We may as well expect a watch to keep correct time when not regulated!

Powdered Turkish, or Chinese Rhubarb taken occasionally in small quantity, will be found an excellent restorative, in producing activity in that organ. It also purifies the blood and benefits the kidneys.

Some physicians say, Rhubarb only acts on the stomach and is productive of no real benefit to the blood. The contrary is the fact, Rhubarb enters the entire system through the blood. By rubbing the hands briskly together, a few hours after using it, you can distinguish, very perceptibly its odor.

Even persons in good health would be benefitted by using this harmless vegetable regulator at least once a month.

Effects of Over Eating. — Excessive indulgence in the pleasures of the table, has hurried more people to the grave than war, pestilence, famine and alcohol combined ! War may ravage a country for a brief period, but many years of peace and prosperity will succeed. A pestilence may waste cities, or even provinces, but after all it touches but a fraction of the human race; famine is unknown in many lands, and the gaunt form of starving want is seldom or never seen in this happy country of overflowing abundance ; the use of alcohol is confined to a class comparatively small.

In contrast with this, behold the work of over-eating ! Its ravages are ceaseless ; from year to year it pursues its work of destruction without pause or interruption : it wastes not only cities and provinces, but rioting throughout the whole broad world, it spreads disease and death among. all classes, ages, sexes and conditions—

maidens and matrons—infants and children—the feeble and the robust, are swept indiscriminately into the grave, by this fell destroyer.

And this over-eating, combined with the exciting stimulating nature of our food, often inflames that thirst which can be quenched only by the stronger fire of spirituous drink.

After over-eating, the greatest error in our dietetic habits is too great variety, and complication, in our dishes. Look at the heterogenous compounds that constitute our modern entertainments! even our " plain family dinners." Here we have meats of all kinds, cooked in every imaginable unwholesome manner, and served up with an endless list of stuffings, seasonings and garnishments : with these, we have pastries and confectioneries and sauces, tea and coffee, hot drinks and cold drinks, sweet drinks and sour drinks, drinks freezing and drinks burning : in short we have a medley of incompatibles that bid defiance even to the subtle analysis of the vital chemistry of the stomach.

With such habits as these, is it strange that women get sick? Is it strange that they die? Is it not more strange that they live as long as they do, when the system is subjected day by day to such outrages?

Many more *would* die did not Nature manage to relieve herself by vomiting, or in some other way.

Our food should be plain and simple; it should have sufficient variety to prevent dissatisfaction, but each meal should consist of but few dishes. *This is a law that can not be violated with impunity.*

Food should be thoroughly masticated; when this is done no inconvenience will be experienced in partaking of a full meal without drink.

There are two benefits to be derived from thorough mastication of food.

I. The stomach will have less work to do, since it will not be obliged to perform any extra labor in reducing the food to a homogeneous liquid, and thereby become prematurely worn out.

11. The food becomes thoroughly insalivated only, when properly masticated.

The saliva is a digestive fluid, and without its aid the food can not be properly digested; therefore let every woman eat slowly and masticate her food well.

As little fluid as possible should be drunk while eating. A celebrated English writer on visiting this country, remarked to a friend that; — "the Americans while traveling, and lunching at a railroad-station, reminded him of the working beam of a steamboat,—when one hand of the traveler returned from conveying food to the mouth, the other was on its way with the fluid."

When we use drink with our food we are apt to wash it down half masticated, and, what is equally as detrimental to digestion, we fill our stomachs with fluid which serves only to dilute the gastric juice, and prevent it from doing its work properly, for the food can never be digested when the stomach contains much other fluid besides the gastric juice.

Thirty minutes is as little time as a person should occupy in eating an ordinary meal. A portion of this time should be spent in cheerful conversation on some pleasant topic ; for there is nothing more promotive to digestion than cheerfulness of mind.

DYSPEPSIA.

Dyspepsia, of all diseases, is one of the most common that afflict humanity, and the suffering is by no means confined to the greatly abused stomach.

The brain at once enters into sympathy with this important organ of digestion when it is disordered. So intimately are the head and stomach connected by the nervous system, that mental disturbances will destroy appetite, and arrest the progress of digestion ; and digestive derangements will produce depression of spirits, instability, hypochondria, and almost insanity.

The direct causes of dyspepsia, nearly every-body is familiar with. They are chiefly — rapid immoderate, and irregular eating ; excessive drinking ; injudicious drugging ; excessive brain labor, grief, and anxiety.

The importance of the salival fluid in performing the digestive function, cannot be over estimated.

The excessive use of alcoholic liquors irritates and inflames the lining of the stomach, and this leads to dyspepsia. Only those who have weak or feeble stomachs without irritation are benefitted by the use of tonics or stimulants, and even then, great care should be exercised in avoiding all tonics, or drinks, which do not stimulate and nourish the system. I consider Lager Bier an excellent and healthy beverage if judiciously used. All lager contains more or less tar, which can readily be perceived if the interior of a recently emptied keg be examined, as the action of the beer causes the tar to settle on the inside of the keg.

This tar is an excellent stimulator and purifier of the kidneys. A moderate use of this beverage will greatly strengthen that important organ. The immoderate use of condiments also induces irritation or inflammation of the lining of the stomach.

I am often surprised beyond expression at the test of endurance some people put upon their stomachs in the wholesale use of pepper, horse-radish, etc.

The amount of any one of these things swallowed at one meal by some individuals, would draw a blister, in an hour or two, if applied to any external part of their persons.

How the stomach manages to dispose of these things without getting burned, is a mystery to anybody who realizes how much more suscept-ible the mucous membrane is to the effects of irritants, than is the cuticle. Hence, it will be seen, that the immediate causes of dyspepsia are as numerous as are bad habits.

The predisposing and perpetuating causes of dyspepsia are, — inactivity of the liver, which causes impure blood, and derangements of the nervous system.

When the liver is at fault, the lining of the stomach is liable to an attack of eruption, or irritation, or inflammation.

In this form of dyspepsia, the invalid experiences pain, soreness, gnawing, burning or
other inflammatory symptoms, with an empty
feeling, sourness, trembling, nausea, etc., at the
stomach. Not all of these symptoms in any one
case, but some one or more of them.

When the dyspepsia proceeds from nervous
derangements, the symptoms are usually, palpitation of the heart, trembling at the pit of the
stomach, a weak or all-gone feeling at the
stomach, while the body appears attenuated, and
the countenance pale, the sleep disturbed, the
spirits more continually depressed, and the
mental and physical energies subdued.

Professional women, teachers, and other brain-
workers, are most liable to that form of dyspepsia
which is perpetuated by nervous derangements.

By too close mental application they exhaust
nervous vitality, and consequently, too little
nervous stimulus is given to the stomach to
render digestion properly active. Dyspepsia of
this form may also proceed from nervous derangements induced by any excessive mental

emotion, or from diseases of the procreative organs, as these affections invariably prostrate the nervous energies.

Dyspepsia, in many cases, is perpetuated by both liver and nervous derangements, or in other words, the liver being out of order, the blood of the dyspeptic is impure, and the nervous forces insufficient or misapplied, a complicated form of the disease exists.

Physically, the dyspeptic has many evils to contend with; pain in the chest and other parts of the body, particularly the left side and the sternum. The muscles of the body become weak and flabby, manifesting soreness on the least unusual exertion, with lameness in the limbs, etc. There is tenderness in the region of the liver, and the spine, felt upon pressure.

In cases of dyspepsia like these mentioned, the patient should take a teaspoonful of powdered Rhubarb, mixed with twice the quantity of sugar, and a little water, frequently. This is the best thing to purify the blood, and assist the action of the liver. Then active manipulation, accompanied by animal electricity, will be found sufficient for the most obstinate cases.

I have annually treated successfully, hundreds of patients laboring under this difficult chronic disorder, whose systems were nearly ruined from the quantity of drugs swallowed.

FOOD FOR DYSPEPTICS.

As to what a dyspeptic should eat! my reply is, eat anything that has the reputation of being digestible food, that best agrees with the sufferer.

No one can select the food for any individual case, so well as that individual herself,—provided she observes effects, and governs herself accordingly; but all dyspeptics may safely and beneficially give attention to one rule, viz., eat slowly—masticate every mouthful of food thoroughly before swallowing it, and take plenty of exercise, but not directly after a meal.

A teaspoonful of camomile tea, half an hour before or after each meal and when retiring for the night, will afford relief, and give assistance toward a permanent cure.

PART III.

EXERCISE.

Girls who are educated according to the rules of " modern society" are ruined in health by the time they leave school.

But should one possess sufficient natural vigor of constitution to resist the destructive influences to which she has been subjected, the work of death is generally completed when she "enters society." She then doffs short dresses, which are exchanged for long skirts, that are anything but favorable to free muscular movements.

She is now denied the little liberty she had in her girlish days, and the small amount of exercise allowed her by the fashions of society, is far from being the best for the promotion of health and vigor.

Exercise on foot is considered "ungenteel" and is taken either not at all, or only when the weather and everything else are perfectly favorable, and then this exercise is a mere listless stroll for a short distance and is unworthy the name of exercise, in comparison with the full, free, natural, unrestrained movements, which bring all the muscles into play, expand the lungs, quicken the circulation, drive the blood to the toe and finger ends, arouse the brain, invigorate the digestive organs, and reanimate all the vital powers.

These devotees of fashionable society, instead of employing themselves in some useful occupation that would give healthful exercise to both mind and body, spend their days in lounging on sofas, or in making fashionable carriage calls. And are these the hope of our country? Are these the mothers of future generations?

If so, the term of human life — already so frightfully abbreviated—must grow shorter and shorter, till the race becomes extinct.

Exercise should be of such a nature as to bring all the muscles into action. If this can not be done by any single movement, the exercise should be varied so as to accomplish this end.

WALKING, when actively performed is an excellent exercise for the muscles of the lower extremities, and if the arms be placed behind the back and the shoulders be thrown backward, the chest may be enlarged while engaged in this exercise.

If young ladies were a little more tom-boyish now-a-days, and would indulge freely in this and other school-girl exercises, their health and happiness would be much promoted, while they would lose nothing in the estimation of sensible people.

DANCING, if it could be practiced in the *day-time*, and in the open air would be unobjectionable ; but not better than walking or running, and especially when the dancing is performed in the stiff, languid unnatural style required by fashion. Ladies should adopt .the easy *non-chalant* style and not lean on their partners while dancing.

Singing and reading aloud are excellent methods of cultivating the vocal organs, and of expanding the chest, provided the lungs are supplied with an abundance of pure air.

But most exercises, when engaged in for the *sake* of *exercise*, are likely to become irksome, and to be "voted a bore." Exercise, then, should be combined with some useful occupation that will employ both brain and muscle.

If young ladies would sweep the house, dust the furniture, work in the garden, and do many things pertaining to good housewifery, they would lose nothing in true dignity, while they would greatly promote health, and be a much more desirable acquisition to those with whom they may be associated with in after life.

It is very unfortunate that the domestic employments which brought health and happiness to the households of our mothers, are considered menial, and beneath the dignity of the daughters of this generation.

Rebellion against the law of labor and the wasteful extravagances which characterize the women of this age, are the reasons why young men "cannot afford to marry," and thus girls marry men in advanced life, who have accumulated sufficient means to "furnish an establishments," but who have lost the vigor and freshness of their youth, and who can never appreciate womanly worth as they should.

RIDING ON HORSEBACK is very good exercise for young ladies and is preferable to carriage riding. It is considered to be particularly appropriate in cases of weak digestive organs ; but I am disposed to think that this mode of exercise has been rather over-rated by some of our best physicians.

My experience has been that more cases of weakness, spinal deformity, disease of the womb, and other organs, are caused by the improper position maintained while riding than by any other method of exercise.

No master should be allowed to instruct young ladies in riding, unless he is thoroughly acquainted with anatomy, and familiar with the evils that arise from a wrong position while riding.

Ladies should sit evenly and firmly in the saddle, as leaning more on one side than the other, will have an injurious effect on the muscles of the spine,—which very frequently causes curvature of that organ.

Children at school should be taught to sit upright at their desks, and not be allowed to bend forward while pursuing their studies.

Those who are in the habit of writing or reading with the body bent forward, are exposed to the combined influence of two causes of deformity and contracted chest, that no constitution can long withstand. These bad positions prevent the full expansion of the lungs by compressing the chest and interfering with the breathing muscles.

Mothers make a great mistake in neglecting to instruct their children in this important matter.

How can we expect teachers to advise children to maintain a correct position at all times while under their charge—which is as important as mental acquirements—when they themselves know so little of anatomy, and "the thousand ills" to which children at school are exposed ?

The Gymnasium, as a rule, is an important item in furnishing patients for physicians.

Very many cases of chronic diseases come under my observation, where the cause is directly traceable to injudicious exercise at gymnasiums.

A young lady should not be allowed to attend a gymnasium unless accompanied, or thoroughly instructed, by the family physician, as to what manner of exercise is best adapted to her physical constitution.

I furthermore say, that no gymnasium should be allowed to exist unless under the direct supervision of a physician, or manager, thoroughly acquainted with physiological anatomy.

MUSCLES.

People generally have a very confused idea about muscles, tendons and nerves. We often hear them speaking of the stretching of the *nerves*, as if these were the cords or pulleys that moved the body. Now, the nerves have nothing to do with our motion, only to convey the commands of the brain to the muscles, which are the immediate active agents of locomotion, and all our movements.

The flesh, or muscular tissue, is composed of

bundles of fibres of various sizes, enclosed in a membrane or sheath. These bundles are composed of smaller bundles enclosed in the same way, and these again of ultimate microscopic fibrils, each enclosed in a very delicate membrane.

All these bundles and fibres are held together by a delicate web-like tissue, and this tissue also lies between the different muscles and the skin.

The muscles are attached to the bones by glistening cords called tendons or sinews. The mere fact of muscle entering so largely into the composition of the system, would indicate to any mind its importance in the physical economy. This tissue constitutes more than half of the weight and bulk of the body. It has but a single function, and that is *contraction*, or the approximation of the extremities; for experiments show that the bulk is unvarying.

By contracting, and in proportion to the vigor of the contraction, muscle is capable of *moving* the bones and other appendages with which it is connected. It also forms the walls of the hollow organs, and by contracting, lessens the calibre of such organs, and impels their contents onward.

The muscles are crowded with blood vessels; the larger trunks of which pass through, and the smaller are distributed within them, for the supply of nutrient matter.

Muscle is visably distinguished from other structures by its red color. The contraction of a muscle is effected by the contraction separately of the fibres of which it is composed. These fibres act only through a portion of their length at the same moment; the contractions seeming to travel from one portion to another of the fibrils, each portion becoming relaxed as the action travels beyond it. Muscular contraction never takes place independently of an exciting cause or *stimulus.* The power effecting this act is derived from the nerves distributed to the muscular structure. These nerves have their origin in the spinal axis, and are also generally connected with the seat of the will. So that impressions received from without the body by the sensitive nerves, and those originating in the mind, are capable of directly inducing muscular action, and consequently motion, in all the organs that are connected with them.

THE EFFECTS OF MUSCULAR CONTRACTION ON THE CIRCULATION.

Muscular Contraction affords powerful aid to the circulation of the parts in which it takes place, in several distinct ways. The effect of the pressure of the contracting muscle upon the blood-vessels that penetrate it, or that are contiguous, is to hasten the flow of the contents of these vessels. The tendency to displacement of these contents can only operate in the direction allowed by the valves of the veins; that is, in the heart-ward direction. At the moment the contraction ceases, the vessels of the part contain less blood ; but the pressure from the arterial side instantly supplies the part more abundantly, so as to distend the vessels.

The benefit derived from these effects on the circulation is by no means confined to the muscles. All other organs connected with the blood-vessels that supply the muscles participate freely in the same advantages ; and it would seem that this is the appointed way in which to secure the nutritive supply in its perfection to the tissues generally.

The province of the muscles, numerous and powerful as they are, seems to be not only to secure their own health by the exercise of their function when in a healthy state, but to minister to the good of all other structures ; for all depend alike for their nourishment upon a common reservoir, whose distribution could not be efficiently maintained without the assistance so largely rendered by the muscles.

The muscles are not only the agents by which we perform all our voluntary movements—they play an important part in digestion, circulation, etc., for the heart is a hollow muscle, while the stomach, bowels, bladder, liver, and other organs are each provided with muscles which do their work without the agency of our will.

As already intimated, the muscles have much to do with keeping the body erect, and in preventing it from falling forward.

The muscles of the spine are the principal

agents in maintaining the erect position, and if these muscles are enfeebled or injured by wrong action or compression, deformity and ungracefulness must inevitably ensue.

DUMB-BELLS.

I do not approve of the use of dumb-bells in the exercise of young ladies. Many of the movements are likely to strain and displace the smaller ligaments and muscles of the spine and other important organs. Some movements may be found beneficial while others are more or less injurious.

The "lift" exercise should not be indulged in. Girls should refrain from lifting either in exercise, or the performance of household duties.

The evil likely to arise from the straining of the muscles and tendons called in play, while in the act of lifting, may result in a serious chronic injury to the spine or of the abdominal viscera.

CASE OF CONTRACTED CORD.

The attention of the reader is called to the following remarkable case, the history of which may prove interesting, though similar cases frequently claim my attention.

A former patient, who knowing that chronic diseases, and cases pronounced " incurable," and where the family physician could do no good, were my specialties, desired me to visit the bedside of a young lady friend who had been confined to her bed for *over three years.*

The circumstances of the case are as follows :

One day, in company with friends, she visited a bell tower, and while there amused herself swinging on the rope used in ringing the large bell.   A sudden painful sensation in the vicinity of the abdominal organs, interrupted this injurious amusement.

She was obliged to be carried home and placed in bed.   A physician was called to attend her, who pronounced it *an injury to the muscles of the spine.*   After an ineffectual attempt to alleviate her suffering—which was intense — by drugs, etc., a consulting physician was called in.   After a consultation, they pronounced it *an iujury of the womb.*

An operation was performed by these doctors, which terminated in no beneficial results, but left the patient much worse ; in fact quite helpless, with a scar three inches long in the left groin.

After a thorough examination of all the cords and muscles, I found that the conclusions of these medical men were entirely erroneous. The trouble was caused by the contraction of the Sciatic cord, which had been injured. This cord extends from the spinal column downward to the big toe, and is susceptible of severe pain when injured.

Under my treatment, by gentle and active manipulation of the muscles in the entire body, a healthy action, and free, full circulation gradually took place, which gave life and vigor to the diseased and strained muscles and cords. Continuing the manipulation, the contraction gave way, and the cord which laid flat and powerless, raised itself and resumed its function. The patient was very soon enabled to walk, and to-day enjoys excellent health, and only recently presented me with a photograph of a diminutive specimen of manhood who calls her mother.

INJURIOUS SEATS.

I would here call the attention of all persons interested in the reformation of prevalent evils, to the palpable injurious effects on women, by the wrong, and uncomfortable construction of seats in our city horse-cars. Most of them,— instead of being straight or slightly raised at the point where the spinal column should rest, which should furnish support for the spine and other organs—are concave or hollowed out in the centre, which, besides being uncomfortable, have a direct tendency to cause falling of the womb, weakness of the bladder, stretching of the rectum, and diseases of the spine.

This evil which has ruined thousands of our women should be abated. These concave seats should be removed and replaced by the more comfortable ones that furnish support and ease while we are seated.

Not only in horse-cars, do we find these

injurious seats, but very often in our houses, schools and churches. Every woman suffering from disease of the womb, or weakness of any form, in the urinary organs, should exercise great care in the selection of seats. A hard firm seat is more conducive to health than a soft cushioned one. The back should not be curved, but straight across and slanting outward.

In concluding my remarks on exercise, I would add that every lady who desires to enjoy vigorous health, should walk at least two hours daily, one hour in the morning, and one just before sunset.

The good results accruing from the regular performance of this duty, will more than compensate for any inconvenience which may sometimes attend it. It will beautify as well as strengthen; it will give light to the eye, rose to the cheek, and elasticity to the movements.

If you are an invalid and walking fatigues you, do not therefore give it up without a struggle. Try walking very short distances, with rests between, and you will probably find that the distances can be increased and the walk prolonged, day by day, until a long walk. becomes both a pleasure and a benefit.

Work about the house is never so good as walking, because it is not done in the open air, still, where the household duties involve much standing upon the feet, carriage riding may be preferable. But if the indoor occupation be sedentary, walk—walk ! It is the only way to keep yourself in good health.

Walking is the one generally available and indispensable exercise, but should never be indulged in *when the weather is foggy.* If women walked more they would suffer less.

HINTS ON DRESS.

THE great law of dress, to which everything should be made subservient should be announced as *health and comfort first, ornament next.* The slightest review of the fashions of the day will convince everyone, that they, with few exceptions, stand directly opposed to health and comfort, and that the latter has been sacrificed through false notions of the beautiful, or through a blind subservience to the decrees of the fickle goddess.

One important law of dress is that uniformity should be observed ; thereby avoiding great and sudden changes.

Here is a young lady who generally has the upper part of her person covered ; but now she is about to attend a ball or an evening party, and fashion decrees that she must wear a "a low neck and short sleeves," her arms and neck are therefore entirely bare, or they have nothing over them except some gauzy web-like tissue which gives no protection at all, and then when the body is debilitated and relaxed, from breathing a heated and vitiated air for hours, and from loss of rest, and when it is reeking with perspiration, she exposes herself to the cold and frosty night air.

Is it at all strange that such gross violations of the laws of health as this should be followed by disease and death ?

This unequal temperature, this exposure of parts usually covered, unbalances the circulation

and is the fruitful source of "bad colds," consumption, rheumatism, etc. And they who thus
expose themselves *must* suffer the consequences.

Many who by excessive dress upon the
chest, make their lungs very sensitive, do not
scruple to remove the dress entirely from the
upper half of the chest and the arms on a cold
night, go to a ball-room and dance all night, and
when morning comes, wonder how they took
cold.

It is often said that the chest can become
accustomed to such exposure as well as the face,
but we learn from anatomy that the face is supplied with an extra circulation to protect it
against its inevitable exposure.

The more a person exists in a hot atmosphere,
the less able does the skin become to react upon
cold, and the more, therefore, does that cold tend
to drive the blood from the exterior to the
interior, and increase the congestion of blood
there.

It is said that all this excessive clothing
is to keep out the cold, but in this most unsteady

of climates the thermometer varies from five to twenty degrees in a day, and can it be said that the same amount of clothing is necessary in both temperatures? On the contrary the very excess of clothing at the higher temperature, renders the skin exquisitely sensitive to lower temperature, which comes on, very frequently, in half an hour.

To keep the skin in active warmth 'by a quantity of underclothing is a most fallacious and injurious attempt. A considerable amount of waste of the body is effected by the skin, and such waste cannot go on without free contact of the atmospheric air, contact which is materially prevented by the mass of garments alluded to.

The consequence is; that materials are retained in the circulation of blood, which ought to be expended at the skin, and, by their retention, prove a source of disorder to the organs in general. For this reason I disapprove of ladies wearing flannels next the skin. It is desirable to avoid all clothing which shall have for view to keep the body in a state of artificial heat.

The skin should be made independent in this respect, its warmth should be the result of the chemical changes actively going on in its actively circulating blood-vessels, and its nerves should be able to throw off, by the reaction of the circulation, those sources of irritation which its subjection to them proves so disordering to the brain and spinal cord.

The clothing should be warm without being burdensome. Many women clothe the body too warmly ; loading it down with skirts, etc., while the limbs are exposed to a constant current of air. No woman dressed in the usual manner, can walk without creating a current of air about her limbs, by the swinging motion given to her dress.

This must of necessity chill the limbs and prevent the free circulation of the blood. The lower limbs should be clothed in proportion to the outer dress.

A point to be considered in adjusting the dress to the body is ; that it should set free and easy and should not cause pressure on any part, or interfere in the least with any movements of the body or limbs.

The chest must be especially guarded against pressure or constriction. If the waist is drawn in there can not be free breathing, and without this, there can be little vitality.

CORSETS BENEFICIAL.

Corsets, to be healthful, should fit the figure perfectly and comfortably.

Too sweeping censures have been passed upon corsets. When they are properly made and judiciously worn, I believe them to be not only harmless but *beneficial*, furnishing needful support and protection to certain delicate organs.

To do this, however, they must be made to fit the individual form ; not bought in furnishing-stores. Many women buy what is called a *handsome* corset, and then fit themselves into it by tight lacing. Harm ensues, and they, or their physicians, blame the corset. They would better employ their time in learning the difference between use and abuse.

Corsets should be made long, coming well down over the spine and the abdomen. No iron or steel should be put into them (unless in the front, and this should not come in contact with the body), but only stiff whalebones; finally, they should close completely in the back, not gap an inch or two, as is the usual custom.

Such a corset will support, and at the same time protect from harmful pressure, either directly or indirectly, the breasts, the waist, the abdomen, the womb, the bladder, and the rectum.

I know whereof I speak, for I have worn corsets from childhood, and I possess to-day an amount of strength and vitality that few women can equal.

I give treatment daily from morning until night, sometimes for three hours, without any rest whatever ; my fund of reserve force seldom fails. Yet if I discard my corset, as I have sometimes done by way of experiment, I soon experience great weakness, followed in time, by pain.

Moreover, patients have come to me with

curvatures of the spine, wearing heavy, torturing supports of iron,—without which, however, they were unable to keep an erect position,—and I have adjusted a corset to them which answered every purpose of the iron, without the weight or discomfort, which they have worn until cured.

Finally, I have put suitable corsets on girls of fifteen or sixteen, who were suffering from general debility,—the muscles lax, the shoulders bent, the organs all more or less displaced or enfeebled,—and they have grown strong and muscular, with straight, handsome figures. Of course there must be no tight lacing : undue compression of the body will produce a disorder somewhere. But there is no reason why corsets should be made tighter than dresses; while they *can* be made to afford more support.

BEDS AND BEDDING.

Permanent injury is likely to result to women, by inattention to their beds and bedding. Feather beds are very prolific sources of disease, and hence ought not to be used. The feathers being animal matter, are constantly undergoing decomposition, which is increased by the heat and moisture transmitted to them from the body ; which causes them to send off noxious and poisonous gasses, the result of putrefaction. These gasses are absorbed and taken into the system, thus causing disease. Spring-beds and very soft ones are also objectionable. They should be as hard, and the bed-clothing should be as light as may be with proper regard to comfort. After rising in the morning the bed should be left open for a few hours, exposed to the air, as it is filled with organic impurities that have passed off from the body with the insensible perspiration.

Beds should always be kept scrupulously clean by frequent change of clothing. Many people have taken colds that have resulted in death, while others have laid the foundation of a life-lasting disease, by sleeping in damp, close rooms, or damp beds. If a room, or bed, has not been used for some time, both should be thoroughly aired before being occupied.

BODILY POSITIONS.

Women while sitting, standing, walking or exercising, should always use care to preserve as nearly as possible, an upright position of the body, keeping the head erect and the shoulders well thrown back. If the body is bent forward, the vital organs are compressed ; and if it is bent side-ways the spine is injured.

Many persons seem to forget that the hips are the proper place for bending the body, and they bend forward by crooking the trunk. As well do many mothers allow their children to form a habit of sitting with the abdomen and stomach drawn in and the spine curved, with the shoulders drawn forward, and the head down. Such children will be very liable to dyspeptic difficulties and lung complaints. They will also become round shouldered and will make a very awkward appearance in society. A crooked person never can look well.

I would strongly deprecate the habit of ladies and children using high pillows while resting, or sleeping. It is far better that people should use no pillows at all, or at most, very thin ones. Many are often injured, and their spines distorted for life by this habit. They whose spines have become crooked by any of these causes should make persevering efforts to straighten themselves by always endeavoring to stand and sit erect. If they find themselves too feeble to do this long at a time, they should change their position frequently.

As a rule, I disapprove of people sleeping together, unless separate coverings are used, for this reason : we all possess different organizations, and the amount of electricity and vitality possessed by one person, will either be less or greater in another. And, as the stronger magnet attracts the weaker, so the person possessing the greater amount of electricity will unconsciously diminish the supply of the weaker person.

In concluding my remarks on sleep, I would

remind the reader that if a sound sleep, uninterrupted by frightful dreams, be desired, the necessity exists for avoiding an over-loaded stomach.

When the stomach has work to do the organs of the mind are only partially asleep, and in this condition a train of thought is suggested by some impression made through the ordinary avenues to the brain. Memory and judgment are active in dreaming as well as imagination,—past events are recalled by a train of association,—and we reason from cause to effect, and often draw conclusions quite correct, as if sleep had not sealed our eyelids.

BATHING.

As ladies are less subject to contamination than "the rest of mankind," they would seldom find it necessary to bathe for the purpose of purification. They, if possible, are more unphysiological in their habits than men ; and they are peculiarly exposed, "as society now exists," to all those influences which result in torpor of the capillary system of vessels, and congestion of the internal organs. For this reason, bathing may be regarded as absolutely indispensable.

While it may not be competent to counteract all the evils consequent on numberless violations of the laws of life, there is nothing so direct and effectual in the removal of those internal congestions, which may be considered the sum total of the maliform maladies to which civilized flesh is heir.

Every house should have a bathing apartment ; but, in the absence of all other conveniences, a quart of water and a towel can be procured at all places, and a general " wash down" or bath of some kind should be frequently taken.

The Cold Bath may be generally applied to the whole surface, or locally applied to some portions of the body, as the hands, feet, seat, etc. In either case the general effect is similar, though the particular effects may be widely different.

Chronic invalids are generally the victims of the falsest notions respecting cold baths. They have become by long habits of effeminacy, incapable of bearing the amount of cold fitted to the respiratory needs of the body. They exhibit the greatest suspicion and fear of the most beneficent designs of Nature. They shrink from the very influence which elicits and vivifies their powers, and so they continue to repress and cramp their already weakened faculties.

The importance of developing to a suitable and healthy extent the *heat-making* faculty is quite equal to that of exercise, and is among the first things to which the attention of the chronic invalid should be directed. The practical effect of such a process is very apparent, and is susceptible of demonstration. The water coming in contact with the warm body has acquired heat, all of which is compensated by increased respiration and increased respiratory effect upon the blood.

In the Hot Bath, heat is imparted to the body, the effect of which is to compel it to take on a reciprocal action and return what it has received, by producing moisture at the surface, to be evaporated.

The skin, under the influence of a hot bath, breaks out in a copious perspiration, this effect following with a rapidity proportioned to the temperature. The effect here described can not long be continued, for obvious reasons, without serious detriment to the organism.

The reader will note an important and radical difference between the effects of cold and those of warm bathing. Cold baths, on account of their effects on respiration, are an agency for the removal from the body of its solid materials; while warm and hot baths, by the effort they assist the system in making to relieve itself of heat, remove fluid and saline matters therefrom. In some cases of disease both of these agents are required.

The skin needs nourishment as well as the stomach. Cold water contains more nourishment than warm or tepid water. If the reader doubts this assertion, the following simple experiment when tried will remove all doubt: take a cup full of water and heat it, after which, let it cool; when cold taste it, and it will be found possessing no taste whatever; all the strengthening and nourishing qualities will have been removed by the process of heat.

No woman in health should fail to take a

cold bath daily, but this should never be employed while the stomach has food in it, nor when
the system is fatigued by exercise ; neither should
it be taken while the body is cold from previous
exposure.

If cold from internal causes, exercise to increase the respiration should precede it, and it
should be, moreover, of very short continuance.
A serious mistake prevails in regard to the proper
manner of taking a bath. The directions usually
are to begin by wetting the head and face. This
direction arises from ignorance in regard to the
true physiological effect of bathing, and of the
condition of the system, for the regulation of
which it is useful.

A valuable lesson on this subject may be
learned by observation of Nature. The dog, cow,
and ox, etc., whom instinct teaches to bathe,
stand first in the water for a while to cool off
the feet, before making a general plunge. Our
feet, even, in spite of effeminate precautions, are
much exposed to the damp, cold earth. The effect
of this is, to counteract the tendency of afflux

of the circulation to the head, which is that portion of the body which employs the most blood and most continuously. To obviate this tendency, the feet and lower extremities should be bathed first, longest, and most. Ladies should remember that all baths below the temperature of the body should invariably be taken by commencing at the feet.

It is sometimes said that bathing or showering the head affords relief, implying an effect in opposition to the principles above stated. In this case the temporary stimulus is evidently mistaken for a permanent effect, and if the observation be extended, the result will be found to be opposite that supposed.

After taking a cold bath sufficient friction should be used to bring on a healthful glow. There is no better safeguard against colds.

For invalids, and in all cases where the vital powers are not sufficient to produce the healthful glow speedily, a tepid or warm bath should be preferred. The special objects are to set the blood into more active and equal circulation, and to promote the insensible perspiration by opening the pores of the skin.

Salt will invariably be found strengthening and beneficial when added to the bath.

EFFECTS ON THE NERVES.

The great majority of women and children, whose sensory surface is so little exposed, are greatly benefited by the stimulation and vigorous tone that is afforded by a daily morning bath. It counteracts in the sedentary the ill effects of warm air confined next to the person by clothing, and for all who are out of doors, is an important means for maintaining the health ; but serious ill effects may, and very frequently do, arise from too much, and injudicious bathing.

The abuse here alluded to, arises from an ignoring of the principles relating to the harmony of function, insisted on in this volune. It will be remembered that *all* impressions made upon the *sensory nerves* are accompanied by a *like action* of the nerve centres situated in the brain, the trunk, and especially those of the spine, which is the seat of the nerves of organic life.

SLEEP.

In fact, without regular periods for sleep, there can be no health, as it is during those periods that the tissues of the body are most perfectly built up. While the individual is awake, they are more or less active, especially the sensory and motor system of nerves. Sleep is simply the resting of the brain from all mental exercise, and the consequent cessation of the nerves from all labor.

The amount of time required for sleep varies with different individuals. Persons who are sluggish in all their habits require more time for sleep than a person possessed of greater activity, for the reason that they sleep slower, that is, the reparation of tissues is carried on with less activity. It is for this reason that a woman of nervous temperament requires much less sleep than others.

In order that we may derive the greatest benefit from sleep, it is essential that it should be undisturbed. When this is not the case, the work of changing the blood into the solid tissues is also disturbed, and consequently, the body is not maintained as it should be. We should endeavor to form the habit of sleeping during the whole period allotted to rest, without waking.

To insure sound sleep no food should be taken into the stomach later than six o'clock in the evening.

We should always retire for sleep with our minds free from care and anxious thought, otherwise our slumbers will be broken. Many persons take their business cares and anxieties to bed with them, and study and worry until they fall asleep. As a consequence, they dream of their business affairs and transactions, and pass the night in a half-wakeful condition, deriving but little benefit from their sleep. The woman who would possess health of body and strength of mind must be regular in all her habits—she should retire early and rise early.

She should also remember that one hour of sleep before twelve o'clock, is worth more than two hours, after.

OUR BONES.

I once saw a young lady whose beauty, accomplishments, and general knowledge, made her quite fascinating ; and yet she was so ignorant of anatomy, that speaking of one of her friends who had spinal disease, she said her friend was " dreadfully afflicted with the *spine* in her *back-bone.*" What lady would not shut herself up and study anatomy for months, rather than make such a ridiculous blunder !

The frame-work of the body, that is, the bones, will first claim our attention ; not because the bones are independent of the other parts, but we must have a starting point. The bones form the basis of the human system,—they support, defend, and contain the more delicate organs. Some may suppose the bones destitute of life, and hardly organized, and not liable to disease and death ; but anatomy explains to us the structure of the bones and shows their vessels. These vessels are full of blood which nourishes the bones. The bones grow and decay and are at times the subjects of terrible disease.

The formation of bone is a very curious process. The bones of the infant before birth are cartilaginous. The bones of young children are soft and yielding ; and it is a wise provision, as they meet with many falls that would endanger hard or brittle bones.

I once saw a woman holding her insensible babe in her arms, which had fallen from the top to the bottom of a long flight of stairs. The mother was comforted and relieved from her fears of a fractured skull, when she was assured by a physician, that her child's skull would bend an inch before it would break.

According to Bell and others, the cartilage that supplies the place of bone in the infant is never hardened into bone. These cartilages have their blood-vessels, and the first mark of ossification is an artery running into the centre of the jelly, in which the bone is formed. This artery carries particles of bony matter, which

are deposited, and a minute speck of bone
appears first, then particle after particle is carried
and deposited, the jelly being carried away by
another set of vessels to make room for the bone.
Thus the work goes on, till the jelly or cartilage
is carried away and bone laid in its place.

You now see that bone is made from blood,
as are all parts of the body. This is the vital
fluid that nourishes and renovates the body.
You can now see why a bad state of the blood
should affect the bones. In order to the formation of *good blood*, there exists the necessity of
using *good food*. As every part of the body
depends on the blood for nutrition, how
important that this fluid be not only perfect
in its kind, but properly manufactured, without
injury to the vital organs. We know that a
skillful workman will, by much labor, make
a pretty good article of poor materials. So it
may be of the blood, whilst the eliminating
organs remain in a tolerably healthy state ; but
it does not follow that good materials are not
better than poor. And, besides, we should

remember that this unnecessary labor is wearing out the vital organs.

It is a truth, that in order to have perfect bones, and to keep them in a state of health, the organs whose business it is to convey nourishment to the bones, should be in a healthy state, and they should have the best materials from which to extract this nourishment. And it is certain, if the vital organs are continually disturbed and troubled by improper substances from which to eliminate nourishment, they will become jaded and deranged, and finally, the whole regularity, harmony and economy of their action will be broken up, and all will go wrong.

There is a sympathy between all the organs of the body, however great, complex, or minute ; if one wheel in a clock is injured, all will go wrong, because all the parts are dependent on each other. Now, if women will abuse themselves, their digestive organs, or the other organs in the vital economy that are laboring for parts of the great whole, they must expect, as a consequence, the derangement of the functions; they must expect disease ; it may be of this kind, it may be of some other.

THE SPINE.

The Spine, or back bone, which supports the head, is a long line formed of twenty-four distinct bones. Each bone has a hole through its centre, and when put together, they form a long tube, which contains and protects the spinal marrow. The bones of the spine are very free in their motions.

The spine is flexible enough to turn quickly in every direction, and yet it is steady enough to protect the spinal marrow, the most delicate part of the nervous system. The atlas is the uppermost bone of the vertebral column, so called because the head rests upon it. Where the head is joined to the atlas, there is a hinge joint, by means of which we can move the head backward and forward, up and down.

Another important bone connected with the spinal column is called the dentatus, because it has a tooth-like process upon which the atlas turns. The turning motion is obtained by means of the tooth-like process of the dentatus. When we nod, you see we use the hinge joint. When we turn the head, we use the dentatus. This tooth-like process is separated by a broad flat ligament from the spinal marrow. It is completely shut up from the spinal marrow by this ligament.

All these twenty-four bones joined together make a canal or tube of a somewhat triangular shape, in which the spinal marrow is contained; which appears to be a direct branch of the brain. The whole course of this tube or canal is rendered smooth by delicate lining membranes.

The spinal marrow lies safely there, moistened by an exudation from the membranes. All the way down the spine, this medulla, or spinal marrow, is giving off delicate nerves to the different parts of the body. There is a notch in each vertebra, and when they are put together, two notches coming together form a hole; through these holes twenty-four nerves are given off on each side of the spine.

Between every two bones of the spine a cushion of an elastic substance is interposed. It is called intervertebral substance, and somewhat resembles india rubber. This substance is very elastic, for though it yields easily to whichever side we incline, it returns to its place again in a moment. This elasticity is of great importance; it enables us to perform all our bendings and turnings, and in leaps, shocks and falls, its elasticity protects the spine.

During the day, these elastic cushions yield by continual pressure, so that we are a little shorter at night than in the morning. And in old age people are shorter than in youth, and the aged spine is also bent forward by the yielding of the intervertebral cushions. Any undue inclination to either side will cause distortion of the spine, from the yielding of this elastic substance on one side, while it rises on the other. At last the same change happens to the bones, and the distortion becomes fixed and cannot readily be changed.

The importance of a knowledge of these facts

concerning the spine will soon be apparent. Just think of a child sitting in a cramped and un-natural posture during six hours of each day, in our ill-constructed school houses, allowed little time for relaxation or exercise, and obliged to hold the head down and study, or pretend to study, when the body is often in excruci-ating torment. Is it wonderful that distortion of the spine, with all the distress and anguish it brings in its train, is so common?

The yielding bones of children are more easily distorted than the bones of older persons.

When the frame is yielding, and the whole system most susceptible of hurtful impressions, children are cramped and confined, and exposed to physical influences eminently calculated to ensure moral and physical destruction.

There are many other methods for procuring distortion of the spine; one is to sit at em-broidery,—any trying sedentary labor may pro-duce distortion. Young people whose frames are hardly developed, and whose bones are yielding, sit much in this manner.

Disease and *Deformities* of the spine have become so common, that it seems to me the votaries of science should be deemed guilty, that they neglect to speak out on this subject, and in such a manner that the community can understand.

The want of common and general information, is a barrier raised between physicians and a certain part of the people ; but if those who are abundantly able to understand these subjects, and to benefit the world by their example and conversation, will but use their energies, they will be instruments of great good in correcting abuses.

I do not think I am wrong when I say that *nine cases out of ten*, of all chronic diseases arise from an imperfect condition of the spine, and I furthermore say that physicians pay less attention to the spine—which is a fruitful source of disorders—than to any other part of our anatomy.   Is this because "drugs" form so little a part of the remedy effectively used in correcting abuses of the spine ?

The application of the *Danish Cure* in the

correction of spinal diseases is especially successful and satisfactory ; and the relief obtained in
these cases is more certain than by any other
treatment. I am constantly furnishing to friends
of the Danish Cure ocular demonstrations of the
good effects of this treatment—effects of a kind
that admit of no dispute. One clearly marked
instance of cure of this kind, in the popular
estimation, is more creditable to the skill and
resources of the practitioner, and redounds more
to her honor, than would any amount of skill
and judgment expended upon the difficult task
of preventing the occurrence of these or other
maladies, or even in curing many other forms of
disease of less conspicuous character.

DISTORTIONS OF THE SPINE.

In considering Distortions of the Spine, it
must be kept in mind how much the muscles
have to do in keeping the body erect and upright,
and in maintaining the equilibrium of the body.

If the integrity of the muscles is destroyed,
they cannot support the spine ; for instance, if

H

the muscles that support the chest are paralyzed, they cannot hold the chest upright; hence that stooping posture so common among young women, who destroy the contractibility of the muscles by too tight lacing. The spine is bent forward, the intervertebral substance gives way and assumes a wedge-like shape, and the spine becomes fixed in a degree of distortion.

It is indispensible to the health of muscles that they be alternately contracted and relaxed. You have all probably noticed that we tire much sooner when we stand for a considerable length of time than when we walk. More muscles are brought into action by walking than in standing; they are thus alternately relaxed and contracted, and this is more favorable than either continued relaxation and contraction. Many have distortion of the spine who are not aware of it.

The following extract is from Dr. Warren's lecture on the Importance of Physical Education. The reader will perceive that I strengthen my positions by extracts from medical men of eminence : — " Causes which affect the health and produce general weakness, operate powerfully on this part, in consequence of the complexity of its structure. When weakened it gradually yields under its weight, becomes bent and distorted, losing its natural curves, and acquiring others, in such directions as the operation of external causes tend to give it, and these curves will be proportioned, in their degree and in their permanence, to the producing causes."

If the supporting part is removed from its true position, the parts supported necessarily follow, and thus a distortion of the trunk of the body. The change commonly begins at the part which supports the right arm. The column bends toward the right shoulder, forms a convexity on the side where the shoulder rests, and thus elevates the right higher than the other. Thus it happens that any considerable projection of the right shoulder will be attended by a correspondent projection of the left hip.

I am aware how difficult it is to have a distinct notion of these intricate changes in the human machinery, without an exhibition of the parts concerned in them ; but it is my duty to present the train of phenomena as they exist in nature ; and I think they are sufficiently intelligible to excite consideration and inquiry.

Perhaps it may be imagined that the cases I have described are of rare occurrence, and that we have no occasion to alarm ourselves about a few strange distortions, the consequence of peculiar and accidental causes. If such were in fact the truth, I would not have occupied your time with the minute details of these subjects. Unhappily they are very common. I feel warranted in the assertion already intimated, that of the well educated women within my sphere of experience, about one half are affected with some degree of distortion of the spine. This statement will not be thought exaggerated when compared with that of one of the latest and most judicious foreign writers. Speaking of the right lateral curvature of the spine, before described, he tells us, " it is so common that out of twenty young girls, who have attained the age of fifteen years, there are not two who do not present very manifest traces of it."

The *lateral* distortion of the spine is almost wholly confined to females, and is scarcely ever found in the other sex. The proportion of the former to the latter is at least nine to one. What is the cause of the disparity? They are equally well formed by nature; or, if there be any difference, the symmetry of all parts is more perfect in the female than the male. The difference in physical organization results from a difference of habits during the school education. It is not seen till after this process is advanced.

The girl, when she goes home from school, is as we have before said, expected to go home and remain, at least a large part of the time, confined to the house. As soon as the boy is released, he begins to run and jump and frolic in the open air, and continue his sports till hunger draws him to his food. The result is that in him all the organs get invigorated, and the bones of course become solid; while a defect exists in the other proportionate to the want of physical motion.

A question may fairly be asked, why these evils are greater now than formerly, when females were equally confined? The answer, in reference to the young females of our country is, that they then took a considerable share in the laborious part of the domestic duties; now they are devoted to literary occupations of a nature to confine the body and require considerable efforts of the mind.

You will readily see that if the bones are not properly formed, they will be bent out of place much more easily. We can hardly insist too much on exercise..

TALL LADIES.

Another not uncommon cause of curvature is, that ladies who are tall are often ashamed of it, (ashamed of their glory)! and continually practice a cringing, crouching, or settling of the body, to lower somewhat its height. The effect of this posture must be evident to you all. Also in those who are even low of stature, the same cause and effect exist.

The present system of education for young ladies is abominable. They are taught to be neither muscular nor frank ; to look no one in the face, to observe a sort of Grecian bend, which is the pink of the mode—a perfect carricature on human dignity and symmetry.

And here I would remark generally, that the present system of physical education lies at the foundation of most of these formidable complaints, and that until parents wake up to the importance of establishing proper habits in children, and of forming a healthy system for them, so long shall they continue to be troubled with physical weakness and deformity.

I herewith present the following evidences of the curability of chronic diseases, and beg the indulgence of my readers while offering a few explanations :

I desire it to be understood that these evidences, occurring where they may throughout this work, are presented mainly for the encouragement of the invalid : my time is already fully, pleasantly, and profitably occupied in attending to a practice as extensive as I desire ;

still, no attempt will be made to conceal the satisfaction I feel in being able to lay before the reader some evidences of the extraordinary success which I have been able to achieve under my system of practice.

Although I have cured successfully and permanently many very remarkable cases, where the patient has been given up by the best physicians of New York City, and whose names would probably be familiar to most of my readers, I labor under some difficulty in presenting these cases, as under no consideration would I use the names of my patients for reference. However, should any sufferer desire to be convinced more thoroughly of the genuineness of these cures, by calling on or addressing me, I will place them in direct communication with the patient mentioned in any of the cases given.

CASE OF SPINAL IRRITATION.

Miss T——, of Harlem, New York City, a young lady, had for five or six years been afflicted with spinal irritation, so much so that the gentle passage of the hand up and down the spine produced a general horror or shuddering, with a snapping of the eyes, and a strange feeling in the head. She had been unable to sit or walk erect, but drooped on one side. The head ached continually, and the mind was always confused and could not endure mental application. The stomach was retracted, the lower abdomen tumid, and respiration short. She had been treated by several eminent men of the profession, but had received very little benefit at their hands.

When I was called to see her I found the irritation extensive and severe. No doubt remained with me but that I could restore her to health. After the second treatment she exclaimed " I feel better," and on resting she said " My head has not felt so clear in a year." After three months' treatment she sat and stood erect with ease. All irritation and uneasiness was gone ; she was afterwards able to apply herself to her studies and various manual duties with pleasure.

CURE OF CURVATURE WITHOUT IRRITATION.

Mrs. B——, of Conn., was a large and fleshy woman ; her form was greatly bent to one side so that one shoulder was much the lower ; her spine was much curved but with no tenderness or pain. The abdomen was full and heavy ; she was unable to walk more than a block on account of great weakness in the back, or giving away in it, through the weight of the trunk ; it falling and pressing out of the axis of the body, the equilibrium of muscular action was broken. So great was her deformity that many considered her a hopeless case. I found the cords and muscles greatly contracted and drawn up. By careful manipulation they gradually relaxed and straightened out, so that finally she was able to walk erect and with ease. At this day few persons would ever suppose her to be the same, who for so many years supported this terrible deformity.

In this case, while cultivating equal strength in the antagonistical muscles, a strong corset was used to partially remove from one side the burden, and relieve the spine from its double load. By relaxing the muscles on one side and by strengthening those on the other, a correct position of the body was obtained.

Miss V——, of Providence, R. I., had been afflicted for years with serious spinal irritation, including the bent posture and all the complicated effects of relaxation and displacement, more especially on the lungs, leading herself and her doctors to apprehend an organic affection of them. The back was quite weak and sore, and could in no wise hold her up or bear pressure with the finger. She gradually grew worse until her doctors informed her they could not cure, but only mitigate her sufferings.

At this period I was called to see her. On taking the case in hand, the doctors' instructions were disregarded by the patient—according to my advice, as being productive of no good,—and my treatment substituted. Within three months' time the young lady could walk about the house, and attend to its affairs. Now she is married, and has two sweet children, and will probably live many more years than she would have done had she remained under the treatment of her former doctors.

SCIATICA.

The Sciatic cord is connected with the spine near the hips; it extends downward from the spine, under the knee, through the calf, and thence to the lower extremity of the foot where it terminates.

Sciatica is a pain beginning at the hips, and following the course of the sciatic nerve. Occasionally it is an inflammatory complaint; sometimes it is connected with an affection of the kidney; but frequently it is a neuralgic or nervous pain caused by poison in the blood and the contraction of the Sciatic cord.

Sciatica can be readily detected by pressing—with the hand—the cord under the foot. When found to exist, physicians often administer morphine, and apply plasters to remove the disease. Morphine frequently produces paralysis, which is almost as bad as Sciatica, and the plasters only remove the disease to some other part of the system.

A want of nourishment in the blood will produce contraction, and this contraction can only be removed safely by manipulation, which produces an elasticity of the muscles, and increases and strengthens the circulation.

CASE OF SCIATICA.

For several years a lady, of forty-eight years of age, had been subject to most intense pains caused by Sciatica, trying in the meanwhile a variety of remedies, but to no purpose. The pain drew the affected limb up, so that in walking she could not put the flat of the foot on the ground ; and it also obliged her to stoop. She had a variety of dyspeptic signs, although want of appetite was not one ; but a swollen tongue, somewhat split, inflamed back of the throat, red eyelids, yellow white of the eyes, and a general want of activity in the skin, bespoke something wrong at the centre of nutrition ; and in that conviction I treated her digestive organs and skin, in connection with the Sciatic nerve.

The pulse was large, but yielding and most irregular ; sleep very mnch disturbed. She had undergone violent medication at the hands of the first metropolitan and provincial authorities, but without obtaining any relief. Between the original disorder and the excessive irritation set up by the medicinal treatment, the nerves were in a most alarming condition. Consequently I commenced manipulating the nerves of the spine and the Sciatic cord very carefully. Gradually the pain grew less and less, and after a time entirely ceased. The circulation became stronger, and the blood was forced into the vessels that had long been dead and powerless. The contracted cords straightened themselves out, and soon the lady could walk erectly and without any pain. Now she is able to visit and receive company ; she enjoys life, and is free from all chance of Sciatica, none of which points she could attain under the medicinal plan of treatment to which she had so long been subjected, but the enjoyment of which she now owes to the Danish Cure.

It is very satisfactory to be able to add to

this case the following letter, received from the husband of the patient in January of the present year :

H——, Conn., January 23d, 1880.

MME. W. D. SCHOTT,

New York City.

Dear Madame :—I am truly happy, at the commencement of the present year, to be able to tell you that, during the space of the last eighteen months my wife has been in the enjoyment of perfect health, thanks to your kind and judicious treatment by your excellent manipulation system.

She has been seventeen years married, during which time I never knew her to be even tolerably well, and latterly she had been growing worse and worse, the severe pains tormenting her by day, and depriving her of rest by night. At whatever place we visited, we were obliged to call in medical advice ; and I may say she had the first in and out of New York, and of London—when we were abroad—that could be obtained.

Some of them attributed her complaint to one thing, and some to another ; there was no end to the application of leeches, blisters and morphine, and her inside was literally inundated with a variety of medicines, till she was visibly about to sink under her complaint. A three months' treatment under your care worked won-

ders, and now enables me to say that she has been ever
since, and still continues, perfectly well, is quite free
from all pain, and is able to walk and sleep as well as
any one could desire ; and our neighbors who knew
her former state look at her with perfect astonishment.
From the time she first commenced your treatment to
the present, she has not had recourse to any medicines
or professional assistance whatever.   I cannot, however, conclude this letter without expressing to you my
unbounded admiration of your skill, and my sincere
gratitude for the very great and kind attention which
you bestowed on my wife's case ; and my earnest wish
is that you may prove equally successful in every other
case that may fall under your charge.

I remain, my dear Madame,

Very truly yours,

HEART DISEASE.

We all know that the reception of a long-
expected letter makes the heart leap for joy, but
if it be sealed with black, it causes the heart to
sicken, and almost cease to beat.   Or if one's
rights are invaded, and we are insulted, it rises in
giant force, and beats with hasty and firm strokes,
that sends the blood to the very surface of the

form, and makes the tired muscles ache for exercise.

If, then, such comparatively *trifling external* circumstances, which have no material connection with the heart, can, through the mind, so effectually modify its action, how much more may internal circumstances of a mechanical character, and bearing directly on the heart, be expected to superinduce very important modifications in its original and peaceful action.

When palpitation of the heart is once originated, no matter by what means caused, there are a multitude of effects or results that we may naturally expect therefrom. The first effect is one confined to, or in the heart itself. In most cases, there is a more frequent and strengthened action of the heart, and in *all cases*, its fibres are laboring under agitation, and a disposition to act which is unusual. The natural result of this on the heart's future action is, that it will tend to an unnatural and diseased enlargement of the heart, and that this enlargement will prove, in its turn,

9

a reacting and perpetuating cause of itself, on the
following principles :

We see, in the cases of the farmer, the black-
smith and the dancer, that the limbs most used
by these different characters are very large and
strong. This is brought about simply by the effect
of exercise, which, through all animate nature,
seems to to be the natural stimulus to growth and
strength. So with the heart; its fibres by their
increased action accumulate power, and consequently growth, while the growth and power will
in their turn enhance again the action.

The heart is a great engine for the circulation
of the blood. Its vessels divide into those which
run into the head and arms, and those which supply the lower trunk and extremities. We know
that the distance to the head is shorter than to
the feet and more direct ; of course, then, when
the action of the heart is increased, the blood
must be sent to the brain in unusual quantities,
and with increased impetus. When we recollect
that the brain at all times so completely fills the

cavity of the skull that the very courses of the blood-vessels are imprinted deeply upon it, we can but expect that this surcharge of blood must be attended with some material consequences. Seeing that the cranium is formed of bone and is inelastic, what will be the effect of ejecting in this forcible manner the blood into the delicate organs that already fill the cavity that contains them ?

The nerves of seeing, hearing, tasting, smelling and feeling must be compressed, and there must ensue a sense of fullness and tightness in the head, giving rise to that beating which is felt in fever and head-ache on laying down, in nervous people; also accounting for the relief produced from a straining sensation in the head by the application of a napkin around it.

But for the other morbid manifestations. We may see the soft brain, its fibres and muscles, compressed in every direction. Of course the optic nerve will be in some degree compressed. The nerve affording the ear a medium by which to convey sounds to the brain will be compressed or collapsed, probably both in alternation. The same may be said of the nerves of smell and taste.

Now we know that such a patient will often suddenly, after reaching or stooping, carrying a weight, or ascending a flight of stairs, complain of dizziness, blindness, or confused vision, unnatural and frightful objects, will reel and stagger, holding upon the nearest object for support. The patient often imagines this to be a fit ; complains of a sensation as of water in the head ; of ringing in the ears, with a confusion of ideas and loss of memory ; clasps her head with her hands, and remains in a fixed attitude. When the fit has passed over, she invariably will say that she first felt a sensation of creeping up the spine, the sensation entering the brain and spreading out in every direction.

Sometimes this affection passes off quietly, the patient moving gently and looking around ; at other times it is immediately succeeded by bursts of tears and sobs, the patient not being able to cease or assign any reason for this conduct. At other times they will scream, seem delirious, and talk incoherently.

Such patients will be often telling that life is a burden ; that they have no comfort ; they will be ever looking for death, and yet when it seems to be approaching, will be filled with terror.

Much may be learned from the above connection of causes and consequences. First, we may learn that the cause of palpitation of the heart, as well as all nervous troubles, does not arise from a diseased heart, or any affection of the truncal organs, but from a local muscular relaxation, or general weakness of the nerves employed in conveying the blood to and from the heart, and, as all these nerves and muscles are connected directly with the spinal marrow, it is safe to infer that *all* chronic diseases of the heart originate from some disease of the spine.

In the second place, these diseases do not exist in the imagination or fancy, and do not depend upon a strong or weak mind, neither are they under the control of the most powerful intellectual influences.

. In the third place, the patient is advised to refrain from all drug medications. In disorders of this kind, poisonous drugs will not give strength to the muscles, life and health to the nerves. What is needed most, is judicious exercise for strengthening the muscles and nerves, whose vitality has been impaired, and in order to be able to know which parts most need strengthening, only such a person should be employed who possesses a most thorough knowledge of anatomy, and is acquainted with the location of every muscle and cord in the human body.

This fact constitutes the most important feature in the application of the Danish Cure.

LUNG AFFECTIONS.

Lung affections are very much under the control of discipline. A contracted chest, whether hereditary or produced after birth, is a general precursor and accompaniment of consumption. This difficulty can be greatly, if not entirely, removed. A contracted chest can be expanded. Indeed, we can almost make our own lungs.

When the chest is deficient in space, the lungs are compressed and irritated, and they are unable to inspire as much air as is necessary to properly oxydize the blood and prepare it for arterial circulation.

When the blood which comes into the heart from the veins is thrown from the heart into the lungs, it contains a surplus of carbon—the basis of charcoal. Here it comes into contact with the air inhaled by the lungs, takes a portion of oxygen from the atmosphere, and gives off its excess of carbon. Here, then, the blood, by becoming oxygenized and decarbonized, changes its color ; and returning to the heart, is carried to every part of the system to supply its nutrition. It is then returned again through the veins, to the heart and lungs. Before entering the heart, however, it meets with the nourishment of our food, carried through the thoracic duct into the circulation ; this being added, the blood again enters the heart. In this way the whole system is furnished with nutrition.

The oxygen, taken in through the lungs,

together with a portion of electricity, is carried and distributed to all parts of the body, to maintain its substance and vitality. Hence the importance of having not only wholesome and well oxygenized air to breathe, but a good set of lungs to perform the process of breathing.

If the chest is contracted, the lungs have not room to expand and receive a sufficient amount of air, and the vital powers become impaired. The blood is returned to the arteries imperfectly oxygenized and electrified, and the whole system suffers ; general health becomes impaired, the lungs themselves then often become irritated and inflamed, and death by consumption ensues.

A full chest, therefore, becomes an important matter. If the chest is too narrow and flat, a discipline must be gone into in order to expand it. With proper effort, the chest and the compass of the lungs may be greatly enlarged. In this way consumption may be prevented. Even if it has already reached its premonitory symptoms it may be averted ; or even in any stage short of ulceration, it can be cured.

The manner of doing this consists first in standing erect. Persons with weak lungs are inclined to bend over their chest, letting the spine curve between the shoulders till the lungs become flattened and depressed.

Let every such person bring their mind immediately to bear upon the consequences of this state of things, and determine to stand erect ; let the front side of the body measure as much from the highest point of the head to the feet, as the back side from the same point. Let them also lie straight in bed, with shoulders elevated by an inclined plane, and head lying on the same line of elevation, with a single pillow. This unvarying erectness of posture will of itself accomplish much in relieving oppressed lungs.

A second step to be taken consists in often inhaling large draughts of air, distending the lungs as much as practicable. By continued practice the lungs will be made to contain more and more air; the air-cells become expanded. This should be done many times a day until relief can be obtained.

A third step consists in repeatedly — many times a day—throwing the arms and shoulders back. This may be aided by weights in the hands.

The shoulders should be kept back, and not permitted to curve round the lungs. If such be the degree of debility that the shoulders cannot be kept back, or in cases of children who cannot remember to do so, put on a shoulder brace. But where Nature is able to sustain herself in this process, she will ultimately do better without a brace than with it. Those who use them are apt to depend on them, without trying to discipline themselves. If people will bear this matter in mind, and can possibly support the effort, let it be done without a brace ; do the same in respect to this, as ought to be done in respect to *medicines ;* use them as a last resort, where Nature cannot perform her own work alone.

CURE FOR COUGHING.

Where a cough exists, this will demand attention. One of the best cures for cough is to *stop coughing.* Instead of allowing it to have full sway, increasing the irritation of the lungs and bronchial tubes, let it be suppressed as far as practicable. This will diminish the irritation of the lining membrane of the bronchial tubes and the substance of the lungs. The less the coughing allowed the less the inclination to cough. When this effort can not succeed, then some resort must be had to palliatives in the form of remedial agents. When this shall be done let the mildest palliatives be used which are able to give relief, and use no opiates.

In all cases where a cough is the result of consumptive lungs induced by dyspepsia—and such cases are not a few—the best cough-drops in all the world are made by dropping the habits from which the cause originated.

Another important matter is living and sleeping in apartments well ventilated.

VENTILATION.

Every apartment of a house, and every school-room and public hall, should have a ventilator at the top of the wall.   This allows the air in the room to keep itself pure.

A portion of the oxygen being taken up by the lungs, and carbon being given off by them, the air becomes devitalized and unfit for being received again in the lungs. This impure air being lighter than healthy air, rises to the top of the room, and will pass off if it can find vent, leaving room for pure air to come in.   In this way the lungs are receiving new and healthy air by every inspiration.

For the same reason no one should sleep without free access to a change of air. The offensive smell of sleeping rooms in the morning is owing to the repeated breathing of the same air, till its vitality has become destroyed, and the impure exhalation from the body pent up in a close room, where the air can not renovate itself.

It is all folly for people to talk of being so feeble that they cannot bear a window open,—especially in summer, in the night. Every one can bear air enough to sustain healthy breathing ; and all notions to the contrary are foolish and wicked.

In small rooms, a window, or door, or both, should be opened in winter, as well as in summer. If we breathe the same air twice, it cannot the second time furnish sufficient oxygen for the blood.

If people would give heed to these facts, they would prevent and even cure a large proportion of consumptive cases which appear among us. The strength and endurance of the whole system depend, in a very great degree, on the amount of healthy air that is breathed.

There is great damage done at the present day to the health by hanging under-dresses upon the hips. This unnatural weight injures the spine, and all the other viscera of the abdomen. It drags them downward from their proper location and connection with the stomach, diaphragm and lungs. This leaves a space between these organs which gives a sensation of faintness and sinking at the pit of the stomach. This, in turn, leads often to a bending over of the chest and flattening of the lungs. Other organs also suffer.

The liver is pushed downward from its proper

position and rendered torpid. The bile, which is the appropriate stimulus for the bowels, becomes deficient ; the bowels become sluggish and costive ; and the blood is left impure because the bile is not properly taken up, as is shown in the countenance.

If ladies would have health and a pure, clear skin, they must allow their lungs to receive the air freely, their liver a chance to cleanse the blood, and their bowels an opportunity to clear themselves.

Unless they do this they cannot long maintain a clear skin and a healthful feeling. Costive bowels alone are ruinous to a healthful body and a cheerful mind.

This state of bowels is very frequently produced by an inactive or sluggish liver, also by the whole viscera being pressed downward upon the lower intestine, and preventing its proper action by mechanical pressure.

All other kinds of costiveness can be greatly overcome by discipline in mind and diet ; but that which is caused by mechanical pressure cannot be cured till the pressure shall be removed.

The use of physic in such a case would be as unphilosophical as taking an emetic to get rid of tight boots.

The bowels and other organs which are fallen down upon the lower bowel must be pressed upward. Every weight must be removed from them and the bowels repeatedly pressed upward. If their drooping cannot be overcome in this way, manipulation should be employed in strengthening the muscles of the entire abdomen. A few applications by an experienced person will restore the muscles of the abdomen, which have become weakened by continual pressure, to their original strength.

But where costiveness depends alone on the sluggish action of the bowels themselves, it can be overcome by mental discipline. The mind should be brought to bear every morning on their action. They should be brought under the magnetism of thought. Let the mind electrify the bowels till they will move.

A regular, systematic discipline in this way has overcome many a case of obstinate costive habit. A mental determination, persevered in, will sometimes effect that which never can be done with medicine.

Another complaint prevalent at the present day, is depression and contraction of the uterus. This is generally caused by a weakness in the ligaments and muscles which suspend it, or by a falling and pressure, as already described, of the bowels.

Where it is produced by the latter cause the remedy is obvious. Raise the bowels up to their place, and by manipulation, continue strengthening the muscles till Nature shall again be able to support herself ; for, without this kind of relief in the case, there can be no cure of this uterine derangement.

Here let every young lady see how liable she is to incur immense suffering by the weight of heavy skirts hung upon the hips, and resolve never to run the risk of ruining herself for life in this reckless way. The Bloomer costume is cer-

tainly to be commended for one of its character-
istics,—all the skirtings are hung upon the body
of the dress. This lets the shoulders carry the
weight of the whole dress, and the bowels and
other organs are left free from pressure.

Where depression or contraction of the uterus
is owing to debility of the muscles and ligaments
sustaining it, means must be resorted to for the
restoration of tone. This may be done by giving
tone to the muscular system in general ; for these
difficulties are generally found in those of feeble
physical forces. Hence, restoring the general
tone of the muscular system will give tone generally to this part.

The parts of the system which can be exercised with the greatest advantage in these cases,
are the arms and chest.

Instances have frequently occurred in my
practice, where ladies laboring under this form of
complaint were so feeble, that they were almost,
and sometimes quite, unable to walk.

Many such I have cured by a process of exercise which only called into exertion the muscles

10

of the arms and chest. By sitting and lifting weights, and other such measures of discipline as were proportioned to their strength, many have been restored by me to perfect health and soundness.

Millions of females in this country are suffering from want of some vigorous employment of their physical energies. They do not go out enough in the open air, expand their lungs and exercise their limbs.

Could I impress sufficiently upon the minds of my American sisters the importance of these facts — thereby causing them to augment the hours devoted to exercise and physical improvement—thousands would annually be saved from a consumptive's grave.

The Danish and English ladies generally could take one of our puny, pale-faced American ladies in their hand and carry them through town in their fingers. But walking, though being excellent exercise, is not sufficient ; it only uses the muscles of the lower limbs.

The most important parts of the system to be

exercised, in any one of sedentary habits, or possessing lung affections, are the arms and chest.

For these, some vigorous exercise for the muscles of the arms, chest and abdomen is needed. Raising the tone here, will by sympathy raise the tone in other parts.

DISEASES OF THE LIVER.

The liver is the largest organ in the body and is subject to a great variety of chronic, as well as acute, disorders. It is commonly called the regulator of our system, yet more frequently do we find that organ requiring our attention than any other.

The office of the liver is to suck up from the blood those properties which constitute bile, and to send them to the duodenum to assist digestion, and then to the intestines to lubricate and soften the excrementitious matters, and conduct them through the serpentine intestinal canal.

Torpidity is one of the most common derangements to which the liver is subject. This is the result of nervous disturbances. Either the nervous forces are unequally distributed among the organs, or there is an insufficient supply of nervous vitality in the system. In either case, the liver lacks nervous stimulus, and the organ may be said to be partially paralyzed.

Grief, fright, dissipation, or some bad habit, may produce an unequal distribution of the nervous forces among the different organs of the system.

I often meet with cases wherein there is too great an expenditure of nervous force upon the heart, producing too rapid pulsations, or palpitation, while the liver is almost deprived of it. Other organs may sometimes receive an excess at the expense of the liver.

When nervous debility exists, or when the patient is unconscious of any such debility, and the system does not contain its ordinary supply of nervous vitality, with which to keep the various vital organs active, Nature, ever disposed to avoid greater evils, is apt to withdraw a portion of the nervous stimuli from the liver ; for the reason that no one of the other vital organs could be slighted with the same impunity.

Partially deprive the heart of the nervous

forces and its pulsations would become so feeble that death would soon ensue. Partially deprive the lungs of them, and respiration would become difficult. The patient would gradually die of suffocation.

Partially deprive the kidneys of them, and the secretions of the urine would be retarded, speedily followed with dropsy or something worse. Digestion of food in the stomach must go on, however imperfect, or the system wastes for the want of nourishment, and nervous force must be supplied in abundance to stimulate the digestive process.

In brief, the partial withdrawal of the nervous or electrical forces from any other vital organ than the liver, would be followed with more dangerous consequences. Still, Nature will not deprive the liver of its due share of nervous stimuli, without giving notice at the same time to the invalid. She paints the face yellow with the bile which the liver fails to secrete from the blood. She constipates the bowels, and in some cases, to urge proper attention, she inflicts a painful and annoying difficulty in the rectum called piles.

While thus urging the invalid to give her means whereby to relieve the liver, she often gets insulted with a dose of calomel. She asks for bread and gets a stone. But she graciously pockets the insult, knowing that it is the result of ignorance, and applies the nervous force, generated by the contact of the mercurial substance with the gastric juice or acid of the stomach, to the stimulation of the liver.

Dame Nature is then pestered to know how to get rid of the mercury, and, in some cases, allows it to attack some muscle, bone or nerve, in order that the pain resulting therefrom may drive the victim to efforts to get rid of it.

Although Torpid Livers are found everywhere, they are more common in warm, or newly-settled localities. Says a popular writer: " I scarcely ever examine an invalid from the South who has not a dead liver. My theory for this is, that in tropical latitudes, in consequence of the expansion of the air by heat, less oxygen by weight is inhaled, and that consequently there is not so much oxygen, or electricity, imparted to the system through the medium of the lungs, as in colder climates, while at the same time, the blood is less decarbonized, leaving more for the liver to do.

Under such a climatic influence the system is apt to become deficient in nervous vitality, and overloaded with carbon, unless the habits of the people are good.

Proper attention to diet and other habits would, in a majority of cases, avert such a tendency, but our friends in hot climates like living up to the northern epicurean standard, and not unfrequently absolutely exceed it.

Thus an excess of work is given to the liver by the use of too much carbonaceous food, and less nervous force is supplied by respiration to enable it to perform the labor.

Considering then, that the liver has to filter out a great share of impure and gross matter, it can readily be seen why, at least, those living in climates predisposing them to inactive livers, should exercise great care in the selection of their food.

Instead of being more careless in their diet, the inhabitants of warm countries should be much more careful than those living in colder climates, so that by preserving a healthy liver this organ may do part of the work usually given to the lungs.

People living under a Southern sun can do this with care and the exercise of a little self-denial. Their food should be nutritious rather than stimulating. Gluttony and dissipation above all things should be rigidly avoided.

Remember that the golden rays of the sun may paint the complexion brown, while every organ is faithfully performing its function, but that when Nature brings in a tint of yellow, the liver has failed in the performance of its duty.

There are a great many diseases of the liver which often assume a chronic character, among which are Inflammation and Enlargement of that organ.

These diseases are attended with more or less cough, headache, pain in the right side, shoulders, and often with swelling over the region of the liver. The invalid is apt to be melancholy, dyspeptic, irritable, sallow, emaciated, costive, and experiencing a loss of strength in the lower limbs.

Constipation is generally a close companion of all derangements of the liver.

The reason for this is, that when the liver is affected the bile is not properly secreted, and when this fluid is withheld from the duodenum, the innutritious is not properly separated from the nutritious matter, while the excrementitious deposits in the intestines become hard, dry, and irritating, in consequence of the absence of the soapy fluid, which, furnished in abundance, softens the matter which passes through the intestinal canal.

EFFECTS OF MERCURY.

Liver complaints of all sorts, which are generally the causes of constipation, and hundreds of other unpleasant symptoms, are usually curable if properly treated.

Mercury often relieves, but never cures a case of chronic liver disease. Even if it were an actual specific, the remedy would be far worse than the disease. The way in which mercury stimulates the liver to action is by its generation of nervous or electrical forces in the stomach, which forces are conveyed to the liver by the nerves conecting it with the stomach.

The necessity for employing mercury in any form does not exist, and women should never allow themselves or their children to be injured— probably for life—by the use of this poisonous agent.

In the treatment of the most obstinate and difficult liver complaints, poisonous mercury is of no avail whatever. In such cases the *causes* should be ascertained. If of a nervous character, or the offsping of diseased blood, as in Torpidity, Inflammation, Enlargement, or any inactivity, a course of treatment embracing manipulation and animal electricity in some form should be em- ployed, if the patient desires immediate relief, and a speedy restoration to perfect health.

The application of the Danish Cure in the treatment of diseases of the liver has been emi-

nently successful. My rational system of manipulation and absorption invariably reaches the
right spot, and many a despondent sufferer has
been made glad with the inspiring effects produced by an external application of animal
electricity.

If proper regard would be paid to the various
ways of avoiding liver affections, which are suggested in this essay, much suffering would be
averted. Those, however, who are already
troubled with such complaints, must resort for
relief to proper remedies, and in haste to get
well, they should not tamper with those poisonous
and powerful preparations, which are so apt to
leave the system in a worse condition than they
found it.

During the many years of my practice, a
great variety of severe chronic disorders of the
liver have been brought to my notice. I have
seen livers so contracted as to be drawn up in a
knot, making the performance of any part of
the duty assigned to them utterly impossible.

Again, I have seen livers that have become

so dry and hardened—from the want of nutritious substances and causes heretofore named — as to become almost ossified and no thicker than a person's finger ; possessing no life whatever.

Physicians frequently give patients quinine, morphine, potash, blue pills, etc., for many disorders of the liver. These poisons only temporarily excite the nerves and vessels in the liver without purifying it. This treatment is all wrong. The liver must be *thoroughly purified* before we can expect any good result to follow. Moreover, the action of these poisons on an irregulated liver frequently tends to remove the disorder to some other organ.

It hardly pays to exchange one disease for another, particularly when it is almost certain that you are going to get the "worst end of the bargain."

DISEASES OF THE KIDNEYS.

The kidneys are two in number, and located on either side of the spine in what is denominated the lumbar region. They are bean-shaped, and of a brownish red color, and are largely made up of tubes and cells, and of membrane of so thin a texture, that as the blood passes through the kidneys, the watery portions pass through the membrane as readily as water passes through muslin. It then trickles down through tubes to little reservoirs in the kidneys, and from thence through the little canals called the ureters to the bladder, which is the great receiving reservoir of the urine.

When a person is in health, the bladder retains the water till it becomes full, or until it is convenient to dispose of it. It empties itself through the uretha, which organ performs the office of carrying off the urine ; it is very short and terminates just above the vaginal orifice.

So closely connected are the urinary with the procreative organs, and so greatly are the latter affected, it is not surprising that the former are frequently the seat of painful and dangerous affections.

In my practice I have a large percentage of cases suffering with disease of a chronic nature, located in some part of the urinary organs.

The most common of these diseases are : chronic inflammation of the kidneys, weakness of the kidneys, Bright's disease, inflammation of the bladder, gravel, etc.

Chronic Inflammation of the Kidneys is generally induced by vascular derangements, and is characterized by heat and pain over the loins, and more or less dull pain in the lower part of the back, frequently extending down into the bladder and groins.

The urine has usually a high-colored appearance, and a variableness in quantity. There is a tendency to soreness on pressure, in the region of the kidneys and the lower extremities, and sometimes actual pain exists.

When other complications exist, these symptoms are more or less modified or changed, and it is usually the case that this disease is accompanied with other disturbances.

Unless produced by contusion, chronic inflammation of the kidneys is generally produced by vascular derangements, and these derangements are commonly the result of wrong bodily positions, and stimulating drinks which inflame and vitiate the blood. The treatment necessary, therefore, is that which will restore the purity and tone of the vascular fluids.

BRIGHT'S DISEASE.

This is the most serious form of disease to which the kidneys are liable. It is characterized by pain and aching in the region of the kidneys, by the passage of urine sometimes highly colored and filled with slimy substances, and sometimes by swelling limbs, retention of urine, very painful passages and intense suffering.

Sometimes the passages of urine are frequent and copious, the patient experiences little pain in the back, but experiences great weakness, and the face beneath the eyes becomes bloated, especially in the morning.

Bright's disease of the kidneys is commonly regarded as incurable, and invalids whose cases have been pronounced Bright's disease, are usually discouraged if they accept the diagnosis as correct.

While it must be considered dangerous,—and even incurable if left *too* long,—I have every reason to hold out hope that it may, in severe aggravated cases, be permanently cured by resorting to proper treatment.

My Uncle who was at the head of the medical profession in Denmark, seldom lost a patient from this disease.

The remedy, exclusively employed by him, was obtained in the earlier days of his practice, by combining the extracts of different vegetables, the properties of which are known to act beneficially upon the kidneys. This remedy being purely vegetable, and containing no mineral poison, is a safe and pleasant remedy, acting quickly upon the kidneys, forcing a passage through the obstructions, and removing all foreign substances from that organ. It can be noticed in the urine a few hours after being used, and because of the valuable properties it possesses, is an excellent remedy for *all* diseases of the kidney.

This specific I have used in this country with

wonderful success for many years, in removing Bright's and other diseases from the kidneys.

Repeated requests have been made by its many beneficiaries for its wide introduction to the general public, but not until very recently have I concluded to accept the offer of a wealthy firm to introduce it on an extended scale. It will shortly appear as " Schott's Danish Kidney Cure," and all female patients suffering from disease of the kidneys, by calling on, or addressing me will receive a sample bottle gratuitously, which will enable them to test its virtues. This cure is no patent medicine, but one obtained from extracting and uniting the properties of different articles of food which are constantly found upon our tables.

BILIOUS HEADACHE.

The liver in health extracts from the blood certain properties which, when collected together, constitute bile, a carbonaceous, soapy compound which, poured into the duodenum, becomes one of the agents of digestion as previously described. When, therefore, the liver becomes so diseased as not to do this, the blood becomes loaded with these bilious properties, and the digestion becomes in a measure impaired.

These irritating matters in the blood visit the head as well as other portions of the body, and coming within sensible contact with the delicate nerves therein, cause irritations which make themselves felt in the form of aches ; and these aches are aggravated by the disturbed digestion ensuing from the absence of the bilious properties from the lower stomach.

The bile in the duodenum is very useful, but in the circulation it is a mischief-maker. Nearly all persons subject to bilious headaches have sallow complexions, which are derived from the influence of the bilious matter in the circulation, and usually, too, they are greatly annoyed with drowsiness during the day, and great restlessness at night, while those who do drop off to sleep without difficulty, awaken in the morning with the remark, that they have slept too soundly and feel uncomfortable in consequence.

Bad tasting and bitter mouth, also frequently

contributes to the discomfort of bilious people; because the blood, overloaded with bile, allows some of these bitter nauseous properties to sweat through the mucous membrane lining the mouth and stomach, as well as through the external skin; and, when the coatings of the stomach are covered with this unwholesome secretion, the tongue usually presents a yellow, furred appearance.

This internal bilious perspiration often destroys the purity of the breath, by its being thrown out with each exhalation from the breathing passages.

No person need suffer from bilous headache. Because it is not regarded fatal, many persons go through life with this discomfort, which greatly disqualifies them from enjoying the freedom and comfort which they otherwise would enjoy did they not thus suffer.

The liver being the direct cause of this offending, the main thing is to restore healthful action to that organ. Nothing will do this so quickly and safely as plenty of outdoor air and exercise.

Walk regularly and perseveringly, and do not indulge in much carriage riding. Skillful manipulation will also be helpful.

NERVOUS HEADACHES. ·

It is very seldom that headaches exist without some liver derangements ; but cases sometimes occur in which the difficulty arises purely from nervous disturbances.

Overworked brain may produce nervous headache, or establish a predisposition to its attacks.

The nerves, as well as the muscles, may be over-strained by over-exercise, and in such cases the result will be an ache or a pain. The sense of pressure is more often experienced in the top of the head than elsewhere, but sometimes there seems to be a sense of pressure throughout the brain.

Persons not subject to neuralgia, or given to excessive mental labor, may in some instances be predisposed to nervous headache. Disappointment, grief, and other excessive mental emotions may occasion it ; using the eyes too much when they are weak or irritable may bring on an attack ; it may be caused by a bad circulation of the nervous forces, or a deficiency of them. In the latter case, when nervous vitality is low, the brain lacks strength and becomes tired by the slightest care or the most ordinary thinking.

For nervous headache there is nothing so beneficial as the treatment described on page 167.

NEURALGIA.

Neuralgia is a disease, the cause of which is little understood by the medical profession, many of whom at this late day deny its curability ; and why ? Simply because they have not been able to see into the science of animal electricity to successfully employ it, in the treatment of the more difficult ills which afflict humanity.

The presence of neuralgia is announced by the most piercing, darting pains, followed with brief intervals of relief ; but hardly a moment elapses after a lacerating pain darts along the course of the affected nerve, ere another shoots forth, inflicting pain equally distressing to the patient.

Neuralgia is purely a disease of the nerves, and may affect any part of the nervous system, although it generally attacks the nerves of the face, jaws, breast, and feet.

It is also caused by an impure condition of the blood, or the presence in the system of some poisonous mineral. Mercury or lead may cause inflammation in any nerve which the impurity or mineral may attack, and when the nerve is attacked by either, so that there is danger of the nervous communication being blocked up, the available nervous forces are gathered up and suddenly precipitated at intervals upon the obstructed nerve, by the efforts of Nature to keep the communication open. These violent propulsions of the nervous forces through the inflamed nerve, cause the sharp darting pains. Nature always attempts to get rid of any strange intruder.

The use of mineral drugs, as a medicine, is also a fruitful source of this affection. Many a person, in consequence of a course of mercury, is ever afterwards subjected to attacks of neuralgia.

How it is that manipulation effects the removal of neuralgic pains—when we so plainly
see that the affection is confined to the nerves—
will be obvious upon reflection.

The restoration of nervous action to the
healthy standard depends on a depression of the
activity of the nerves involved. This effect
readily follows the excitement of manipulative
action. By this treatment the functions of the
outlets of the body are encouraged and waste
matters are dismissed.

Even in obstinate cases manipulation will
prove more useful than medicine, since no other
means is so effectual as this, in dislodging and
conveying foreign matters from the system.

PART IV.

THE HAIR.

ITS FORMATION DESCRIBED.

Every part of the surface produces hair, excepting the palms of the hands and the soles of the feet, but the hairs of the different parts of the surface vary much in several particulars. Over the greater portion of the body they are short and fine, scarcely perceptible in some places. The eyebrows exhibit them of stronger growth and greater length, though still very limited in the latter quality, whilst on the scalp, in their luxuriance and length of growth, they attain their maximum.

Hairs are formed by glands, situated either in the substance of the true skin or in the fatty cushion beneath it. The glands consist of a little sac, at the bottom of which is a papilla, or eminence, and largely supplied with nerves and capillary blood-vessels ; from the contents of the latter the hair is manufactured.

The hair, when formed, finds its way outwards to the surface through a tube like the ducts of the perspiratory and oil glands, lined with scalp-skin.

Into these hair ducts, very frequently one, and sometimes two, ducts of the oil glands open, so as to give the root of the hair the advantage of the softening influence of the oil; a knowledge of which fact may serve as a hint that possibly less pomatum is needed to benefit the hair than is often supposed.

The process of manufacturing the hair, so to speak, is very interesting.

First, a fluid is poured out, or, as scientific language expresses it, is secreted by the papilla from the blood contained in its capillary vessel. This fluid, gradually drying, forms first into granules, then into cells, and these cells are aggregated together into the form of the hair.

The hair thus produced is not, however, of uniform structure, but on examination with the microscope, we find that the cells which constitute it present three different modifications.

In the centre of the hair, which is less dense
than the other parts, the cells are but little, if at
all, altered; collected as it were comparatively
loosely together, so as to form a pith, perfectly
analagous to the pith of a feather. Immediately
outside of this pith, the cells are split so as to
form fibres.

These constitute the chief thickness of the
hair, and give it its strength. Outside of this
again, is another layer of cells, but dried and flattened into little plates, or scales, so that in the
rough, the hair has much similarity to a young
twig of a tree—pith in the middle, fibres giving
it strength outside of this, and a coating or bark
outside of all.

The average thickness of hair is one-three-
hundred-and-fiftieth of an inch. Black hair is
thicker than brown, and brown than blonde, as a
general rule ; though I have seen some specimens
of very fine black hair, and, of course, sandy hair.

It has been computed that of black hairs,
147 grow upon a square inch of the scalp, 162 of
chestnut, and 182 of blonde.

The cells forming the hair contain coloring matter, which gives the tint to the hair. This coloring matter, however, is not uniformly distributed through the substance of the hair, but is found chiefly in the fibrous portion; and even in this it varies in different parts, as if some of the cells were fully charged with the color, whilst others have little, if any, in them.

To this unequal distribution much of the variety in the tints of the hair is owing. Thus an admixture of black cells with white ones gives a grayish hue; reddish cells with white ones, a sandy hue, etc.

The rapidity of the growth of the hair varies much in different persons. It has been calculated that with man the beard grows at the rate of one line and a half a week, or six inches and a half in a year.

On the head the growth is evidently much more rapid; at least under the influence of frequent cutting, if not by Nature.

On the head the use of the hair is most obvious as a bad conductor of heat,—to equalize the temperature of the brain. The eyebrows shed the perspiration from the forehead which might otherwise enter the eyes. Just within the aperture of the nostrils and ears it guards these from the ingress of insects and dust.

To these several others have been added by physiologists, partaking more or less of the speculative, and more or less plausible. Whether, for instance, the hair exerts a continued electrical influence, or whether it plays an important part in the chemical process of the animal economy, I am unprepared to decide ; and moreover, a discussion of these questions would by no means benefit or enlighten, for practical purposes, the general reader. It is, however, undeniable that the removal of the hair has great influence in preserving nervous strength and in relieving severe affections, more particularly those of the head, — headache, vertigo, tenderness of the scalp, etc.

This should make the hair the object of attention and care during any prolonged sickness, more especially if the symptoms point to any affection of the brain and its envelopes.

By the term disease, I here mean any departure from the natural and proper condition of the hair.

Such may occur in regard to situation ; it may grow where it ought not, and thus produce unseemliness ; in regard to quantity, which may be increased or diminished ; in regard to color, losing its natural hue and blanching ; and, lastly, the bulbs may become weakened or affected with some disorder.

Having considered these as far as practicable, I will then advise concerning the management of the hair, which I postpone just now, for a convenience that will probably be obvious.

Hair in Unusual Situations.—As a freak of Nature, hair is often found growing in various places, from discolored spots, called moles. These exist from birth, and may be of any size, from a line in diameter, giving growth to three or four hairs, to that of the hand, or—we know not why—larger.

These are wholly unattended with any painful sensations, but may incidently become very annoying in particular situations. They are more or less unsighly; and when very much so, it may be desirable to get rid of them. This can be done by the knife—a simple operation, and one under favorable circumstances leaving no scar.

It is, therefore, a consideration for the person alone as to whether the mole or the cut had better be endured. There exists a very prevalent notion that they are liable to turn into cancers when meddled with, but I do not see, upon general principles, why this should be, nor have I ever seen or heard of an authenticated case in which it occurred.

The error has had its origin, probably, in the fact that certain tumors of the skin do occasionally develop into malignant affections.

The hair may sometimes extend beyond the limits of what is considered comely. Thus the two eyebrows may be blended into one uniform growth, or the forehead may be lessened in height by the hair of the scalp extending too far down upon it. In such cases the individual should coolly consider whether the deformity is really as great as imagined.

A very important step as a beginning,—for a

reference to others will show that very often
certain peculiarities which, in the abstract, might
be considered as blemishes, in the actual har-
monizing with the general style of feature, complexion, etc., are not only not detrimental, but
are really effective in producing an agreeable
ensemble.

The anecdote should be recalled of the painter
who, desirous of producing with his brush a
faultless female face, selected for his models the
most beautiful individual features that he could—
the eyes from one, the nose from another, the
mouth from a third, and so forth ; but the por-
trait when finished was sadly deficient in every
trace of beauty.

If, however, such consideration does not
lessen the impression that an imperfection is to
be removed, and a razor is considered an unfit
implement in removing it, tweezers should be
used, and with diligence and patience, the hair
may be for the time gotten rid of, and for a
longer time than by any other means ; for all that
is as yet formed is drawn out. It must be re-

membered, however, that the manufacture of the
hair is uninterrupted ; the bulb that forms it still
remains, and this cannot be destroyed without
also destroying the skin in or beneath which it is
implanted.   This can only be done by cutting or
burning out the hair bulbs, in which case the
growth will be effectually stopped.

Too Great Profusion of Hair, or extraordinary thickness and rapidity of its growth, can
scarcely be called disease, though, were we to
believe all the marvelous tales that are told of
instances of this peculiarity, we should have
reason to consider it so, and even a dangerous
one, for among the old legends of this sort is one
of a lady, whose beautiful tresses, the admiration
and pride of herself and family, the wonder of
her country, became the cause of her death.
They grew with such marvelous rapidity, and so
thick, that they expended all her vital powers,
and she waxed wan and feeble as they waxed
darker and longer, and richer in gloss, until she
was consumed in nourishing them.

Without believing all this—which is told by

an old writer with great gravity and earnestness—
we can believe, and indeed have seen instances
in which the hair, by its great thickness and the
warmth it created, has caused much discomfort,
particularly in the way of headache, and, indirectly, disorders of the general system.

The remedy is a very simple one—thinning it
out with the scissors ; that is, inserting the points
of the scissors to the roots of the hair, and
cutting off a dozen or so here and there all over
the head.

DEFICIENCY OF HAIR.

The condition of the hair which, with possibly exception of its loss of color, is of most
care to persons, and for which remedies are most
anxiously sought, is where it becomes deficient
in quantity.

Through all ages the hair has been considered
one of the chief graces of women. Among the
earliest nations, sacred as well as profane, it en-
tered largely into rites devotional, political and
social. Its length, the style in which it should
be worn, and the ornaments that might be used
with it, were all presented to each individual

according to sex and station ; and that it should be shorn or left unshorn, under certain circum-stances—that under others it should be sacrificed, and the manner in which this should be done—were also directed by laws equally stringent and particular.

It has been, therefore, from various motives, beginning with those of the highest devotional character, down to such as arise simply from a desire for personal comeliness, always an object of care and solicitude ; and for the fostering of its growth, the increase of its beauty, and the preservation of its luxuriance, ingenuity seems to have been taxed, from the earliest times of which we have record down to the present day.

It is then to the supply of no new want, engendered "in these effeminate days," that we address ourselves in attempting to explain the causes of deficiency of hair and furnishing a remedy for it.

The first step should be to discriminate be-tween the conditions in which deficiency of the hair occurs.

These are chiefly two ; and though one of

them may pass into the other, yet until that· change is effected, a very different course must be pursued from what would be expedient if the second condition obtained.

In the one, the bulb or gland forming the hair has simply become weakened—is unable to perform its function actively and efficiently. The effect of this is, first, to permit the hair to fall out, or to be easily pulled out—as in combing the head.

Next, instead of replacing the fallen hair with another of the same color, thickness, and rapidity of growth, as its predecessor, the one that follows is often smaller in diameter, paler in color, grows very slowly and is also easily pulled out.

This is the condition which so frequently follows fevers and some other diseases producing great depression of the vital powers, and also violent mental emotion having a similar general influence.

This condition is also confirmed by observing the different conditions of persons as to the growth of their hair, in various occupations, which may require the more or less constant use or disuse of covering for the head.

It will be found that among these, in proportion that the head is left uncovered, provided it is not exposed to other adverse influences, the growth of the hair is thicker, and endures longer.

Women are supplied with a thicker layer of fatty matter in the scalp, which, if not especially intended for that purpose, at least serves, among others, to furnish their tresses with a richer nourishment, and, continuing longer than the same matter in men, preserves for them this decoration much later in life ; and yet, with women, how often do we hear the same remark as to the scantiness of the hair, and the early age at which the defect commences—earlier even than in men.

That this must be the effect of something else than natural causes, the provision just mentioned will show ; in addition to which, we have another in the fact that the thinning and baldness in women does not always first show itself where the fat is first absorbed — on the top of the head—but more often is it seen at the sides.

For this an explanation seems apparent, in the habitual treatment of the hair with cosmetics—particularly greasy substances perfumed with essential oils—and in the style generally prevalent in dressing it.

The most injurious effect of cosmetic is, that it makes the hair very compact, so that, like a man's hat, it increases the perspiration of the scalp, and yet does not permit its escape. A style of dressing the hair which is very injurious, is that in which it is drawn very tightly, not only making it too compact, and increasing the effects just mentioned, but actually drawing out by the roots a greater or less quantity every time the hair is dressed; and, indeed, every time it is subjected to any violence, however gentle, as in putting on and taking off the bonnet.

This particular source of the thinness of hair over certain parts of the scalp seems well understood, and I have often heard the remark, "I must part my hair in a new place—it is getting too thin." The more sensible way would be, not to part it in a new place and merely remove to it the difficulty, but to dress the hair in a different manner ; but of this, more presently.   My object just now, is to show that the principle cause of baldness depends simply upon a weakened state of the hair-glands—an imperfect formative force, a defect in the manufacturing apparatus, depen-dent upon certain causes, that may be removed— general debility following some bodily or mental disease, wearing close, air-retaining hats, arrang-ing it too compactly, drawing it too tightly and thus mechanically thinning it out.

The remedy for this kind of baldness, when the cause of it is understood, will, in the majority of instances, be apparent, namely, laying aside the practices which have led to it, and resorting to proper means of taking care of the hair, to be presently given.

If the source of the defect is due to any of the influences just mentioned—though the cause may have ceased, the hair-glands still remain feeble and inefficient—it will be necessary to resort to some direct appliances to bring back their natural strength and ability.

During a practice of many years, numerous preparations have claimed my attention ; some I have found containing not only injurious, but poisonous ingredients, possessing a tendency to entirely destroy the vitality of the hair-glands ; others have been found possessing greater or less merit, few scarcely without some objection to them, in the damage they are liable to do from over-exciting the organs they are intended to benefit.

But the following preparation, which is now for the first time disclosed to the public, has been used exclusively and with eminent success by me, both in this country and in Denmark, and has invariably been found possessing the necessary qualities for restoring life and vitality to the weakened hair-glands, and producing a new growth of hair, when all other preparations have failed, viz. :

Two tablespoonfuls, pure Cayenne Pepper.
A tumbler of strongest Spirits Ammonia.
Two tablespoonfuls of Salt.
Six tablespoonfuls Sweet Oil.
Put these ingredients in a quart bottle and fill bal-

ance with water. Let it stand for nine or ten days, then strain through Swiss muslin.

Directions for Use.—Saturate a sponge with the fluid, and rub well into the scalp, on retiring. If the hair-glands are very weak, use every evening. Generally three applications a week will be found sufficient to produce the desired result.

This preparation, when applied, produces an electrifying effect, stimulating the glands to new life and strength, and, if impaired, it restores the natural and original color to the hair.

In connection with this preparation, manipulation of the scalp will be found most beneficial in stimulating the glands to form better and stronger hair. In addition to manipulation, which should be used once a day, the head may be showered occasionally with cold water, carefully drying it with soft spongy towels, rather by pressing them upon it, than by rubbing it with them, which would have the same effect as a large hair brush.

With women wearing their hair long, the showering will be more or less inconvenient; and yet it need not be so much so as to deprive them of the benefits of it, which I believe to be great.

The chief tax is upon the patience in drying it, but after a little time, practice will give great . readiness in this, particularly if these directions are followed.

First, separate the wet tresses very carefully, and holding them with one hand near the roots, so as to prevent any strain upon them in the other parts of the process, with the other hand envelop them in a soft towel, and press them firmly in its folds from the roots towards the extremities.

This properly done, will remove all the free water ; and then, to dry them thoroughly, separate the hair into as small strands as possible, and sit with it thrown over the back of a chair.

This will of course take some time and patience, but it is the best way under the circumstances, and the time need not be lost, for it is still available for reading or some kinds of work.

Loss of Color in the Hair.—This may be the effect of time alone, and may also occur at a much earlier age with some than with others.

It may, too, proceed from an accidental debility of the glands, preventing them from secreting as much coloring matter as they should.

The instance may not unfrequently be seen of a young person with a full and luxuriant head of hair, which has lost its color, after severe sickness, or some other such impression.

There are but two methods of treatment where this condition exists—the one to restore the strength of the glands ; the other to let them alone, and simply dye the altered hair.

The latter method I do not approve of, as dyes of any description contain more or less injurious ingredients, which frequently injure the brain.   There are many cases of insanity on record, where the direct cause has been traced to poisons contained in hair dyes.   Dyes are not, however, used solely for the purpose of restoring the previous color of the hair, but they are frequently resorted to with a view of altering tints of hair not considered becoming, particularly those in which a red hue predominates.

The color of the hair is not a sole peculiarity in such cases, but it is generally accompanied by a certain kind of skin—that is, one of a particular color and texture—which can produce nothing but reddish hair.

The eyes are generally colored to match, and, in fact, the red hair is but one item in a harmonious *ensemble*, which is often ruined by altering only that item ; the harmony is destroyed, and whatever grace may have derived from that lost.

Admitting that some colors are very much preferable to others for the hair, it is better to leave the tinting as done by Nature's hand, than to run the risk of destroying the harmony of her hues, and to add baldness to the already existing—so supposed—blemish.

Dandruff is considered by many as a disease, and so it may be when very greatly increased in quantity. It is, however, nothing more than the scales of scarf-skin, which are so plenty in the hair ; because, besides the outer surface of the skin to supply them, it must be remembered that the tube of each hair-gland is lined with scarf-skin, and these linings are constantly undergoing the process of being thrown off.

The proper remedy for dandruff is to strengthen generally the scalp and hair-glands, and· wash the head once or twice a week in soap and water.

The Care of the Hair.—I have delayed until now to say anything about the general care of the hair, thinking that the reader would be better able to appreciate the value of the directions given under this head, after reading what has gone before, and after seeing more clearly the nature of the evils which it is purposed to avoid in bringing common sense and reason—not to say anything of science—to bear upon hair-dressing.

Cleanliness here, as in all other cases, is of the first importance. With the hair, it is to be attained, first, by the comb—one with very fine teeth ; and next, by the brush—each of which should be used at least once a day.

It may seem strange, at first, to have to give directions how these very familiar implements should be managed ; but it is the fact, though few amongst us are unable "to make one hand wash the other," there are many who do not know how to comb their heads ; and, in their ignorance, they frequently do much damage to a fine and healthy suit of hair.

The common fault is, that the points of the teeth are carried down to the scalp, and are there pushed along, ploughing in among the hair-glands, to their evident detriment.

This, French *coiffeurs*—many of whom have really very sound knowledge of, and great skill in, their art—have long been aware of, and often given caution against.   If the object be to cleanse the scalp, a comb is not the proper instrument. It is only suited for removing the foreign bodies, whether they be dandruff, dust, or any other sub-stances that are attached to the sides of the hair, and to improve its " lay."

To do this, it should be inserted to the roots of the hair as nearly parallel with the scalp as possible, and then drawn gently along the full length of the tresses, which, if long and thick, should be held by the other hand, between the comb and the roots, when the former is sufficiently distant from the head, in order to prevent any strain upon the latter.

In this way it does its work very effectually, and does not injure the glands. To smooth the hair and put it into proper position, it may have to be carried along perpendicular to the surface, but this can be done without pressing it in too much. For the same reasons the brush should not be used too forcibly or with too much pressure.

To cleanse the hair, there is nothing better than borax, soap and water. The soap, of course, should be mild, and well and plentifully rubbed in, and afterwards thoroughly removed with an abundance of water. The frequency with which this process should be repeated will depend upon the individual—persons with light, thin and dry hair will require it more seldom than those with thick hair, or who perspire very freely.

Once a week could scarcely be deemed too troublesome when the object in view is considered; and this may serve with most, though those in whom the last mentioned qualities of hair are very marked would benefit by a more frequent resort to it.

There exists a popular impression, though I know not to what extent, that water rots the hair, and its too frequent use makes it harsh and coarse. Principles must never be adduced from solitary or occasional cases, which may be deceptive. Frequent wetting of the hair will not rot it unless it be improperly dried; care should be taken to thoroughly dry the hair after each wetting.

Pomades should be used as sparingly as possible, and only when necessary on account of some real imperfection of the hair, such as a roughness or too great dryness of it.

Some women imagine the roots require frequent annointing, that the hair may grow more freely. This is a mistake; clogging up the pores with heavy oil is not the way to promote a healthy condition of the scalp and its appendage.

As to " Bandoline "—a sticky liquid made of gum tragacanth, and used to make the hair lay smooth and look shiny—it is a dirty, clumsy compound, and should be entirely discarded. If the hair is so unruly as to require that it should be glued down to make it submit to a certain style, surely a lady's taste and ingenuity could contrive some other way of dressing it in which this quality will be of no disadvantage, and thus save her head from becoming a receptacle for sour paste.

PART V.

THE TEETH.

The importance of the teeth, and, of course, of their preservation in good and sound condition, though it has forced itself upon all, in some bearing or other, is appreciated by few in its full length and breadth.

Some seem to consider them only as ornaments; others take a purely utilitarian view in regarding them solely as food-grinders, ignoring their other functions, and being unaware of the influence that they may have upon the general health.

The lowest value of the teeth is, undoubtedly, that they possess as ornaments, but this I do not consider trifling.

The next value they possess is as auxiliaries to the organs of voice. Cicero asserted that the teeth tended to heighten the effect of every feature, and modulated the voice to that degree of perfection which no musical instrument could ever attain. The influence of defective teeth upon enunciation is too well known to require more on this head.

Their use as masticators is a very obvious one; yet habits so frequent as to be deemed by some a national characteristic, have greatly discarded them in this capacity; and the impunity with which this is done by many, for the first half of their life, has made them shut their eyes to the possibility that a time may come when the stomach will rebel against doing double duty, and refuse to do even its own proper share if the teeth have not first done theirs.

The fact is, that that part of the function of digestion accomplished between the lips and throat is a very important one, and does not consist simply of mastication, though this is a necessary portion of it, and one without which the others would be imperfectly performed.

As soon as the morsel is received within the lips, the salivary glands, opening into the anterior part of the cavity of the mouth, commence pouring out their fluid.

This is the first and most delicate solvent to which it is submitted. The solid must be broken up thoroughly, and in doing so the saliva is mixed intimately with it, each new surface exposed by the cutting of the teeth being bathed with a fresh supply, which the next moment, by their grinding action, is thoroughly incorporated with it. .

In this manner, not only is the whole mass softened and rendered more susceptible to the influences of any coming agent, but it already has one mixed with it, and from that moment at work upon it.

How different from the same aliment introduced into the stomach without such preparation —when the gastric juice is the sole agent to act upon it, and it has to operate upon the substance still in all its original density, a condition best suited to enable it to resist the impression of any solvent.

Having thus shown the value of the teeth, and their importance in connection with the digestive organs, sufficient insight will be given into their structure and arrangements to enable the reader to appreciate directions for their care.

Description of the Teeth.—The teeth are divided into three parts : the body or crown, that part which projects beyond the gums ; the neck, a slight depression around the body, where the edge of the sockets clasp it ; and the fangs or roots, the parts inserted into the sockets.

The body varies in shape with the purpose for which the tooth is intended, thus it is flattened and sharp at the free edge in the front teeth intended for cutting, but presents a broad and rough surface, instead of this edge, in the back teeth, intended for grinding.

The roots also vary, with the first mentioned there being but one to each tooth, whilst the latter have two and three.

STRUCTURE OF THE TEETH.

Teeth are composed of two different substances, the roots and body of a species of bone, though much harder than any other bone in the body ; and the latter is covered with a still more dense substance, called the enamel—by far the hardest of all animal tissues.

The object of the enamel is to present a very hard and resistant material, and one which will not soon wear out, to the various foods subjected to the process of chewing. With a similar intent, it is used similarly entering into the structure of knife-blades, or hammer-faces. Were all the knife, or all the hammer, steel, the instrument would be too brittle ; were it all iron, too soft.

The one, therefore, has a strip of steel along the edge—the other, a piece covering the part which receives the force of the blow. So with the teeth ; were they all of enamel, they would be too brittle, of bone, too soft, and soon wear blunt and smooth.

To gain each excellence in its proper proportion, the enamel covers all the part of the tooth exposed beyond the gum. Within the tooth is a cavity filled with a nervous pulp, very highly sensitive, and under the influence of injury, exposure, and disease, affording one of the sources of "tooth-ache."

The roots of the tooth are surrounded by a membrane, a similar one to which lines the socket into which they are planted.

Inflammation in these membranes is another source of tooth-ache. They become filled with blood, but cannot expand, and consequently compress the nerve with a power, almost, of a hydraulic press, causing most exquisite agony. A continuance of the inflammation is accompanied with formation of matter, abscess, perforation of the bone, and other troubles.

The enamel of the teeth does not grow; and the first teeth being small, to suit the wants of infancy, they must be gotten rid of, and replaced by larger ones.

It is with this view that, at a certain age, the roots of the teeth are absorbed, the teeth becomes loose, fall out, and are replaced by corresponding ones of a larger and stronger make, to which are still further added, as life advances, more grinders — the last of which are called wisdom-teeth.

In this rearrangements of the teeth, they

are very apt to become crookedly set ; and, if neglected, to produce a very unpleasant deformity through life — often affecting articulation considerably—causing great trouble in keeping them clean—inefficiency in chewing and other inconveniences, all more serious than at first might be supposed.

The importance of remedying any such deformity cannot be too strongly impressed upon the minds of parents, many of whom neglect all attempts at relief, either from ignorance that it can be given, or that it is worth while to obtain it.

The gums, which, in health, embrace closely the neck of the teeth, are of a firm, dense structure, and covered with what is called the mucous membrane. When it covers the gums, this membrane is tougher and denser than elsewhere, for the obvious purpose of resisting the effects of any hard substance pressed against them in chewing.

TARTAR.

In various parts of the mouth, on and under the tongue, in the walls of the cheeks, etc., there are various apertures discharging fluids formed by glands situated in the neighborhood. Some of these fluids are mucous, intended chiefly for keeping the lining of the throat soft and moist, so that the food may pass down easily.

These fluids contain earthy salts, which are deposited upon anything with which they may be in contact, whether it be the teeth or metal used in the construction of any dental contrivance.

This deposit is commonly called the tartar of the teeth; and permitting it to accumulate is one great and very common source of decay of the teeth, retraction of the gums, with exposure of the neck of the teeth, spongy gums, bad breath, etc. ; though in some cases, it is true, the existence of too much tartar, and the other affection, may be the joint effect of some derangement in the general system, more particularly of the stomach or liver.

THE CARE OF THE TEETH

The above is sufficient of the teeth, together with what must be already well known, to enable

the reader fully to appreciate directions for the
proper care of them.

Cleanliness holds the first rank. Teeth in
want of it suffer from two sources; one of these
has already been mentioned, the accumulation of
tartar. Where this has, by neglect, or unavoid-
ably in sickness, already collected, no time should
be lost in having it removed by a dentist, who is
provided with instruments by which it can be
done very thoroughly, and, if with proper skill,
without injuring the enamel.

The gums will then generally return of themselves to the neck of the tooth from which they
have been separated, but if not disposed to do
so, may be stimulated by an astringent wash.
Tincture of Myrrh will be found the best for this
purpose.

The other source of detriment to the teeth,
resulting from uncleanliness, is decay, the most
common and serious affection to which they are
subject. The decay invariably commences at
those points where foreign bodies, whether the
secretions of the mouth or food, are apt to accumulate—namely, between the teeth, or in the

deep depressions in the grinding surface of the
molars, which are prone to become impacted
with food, and very difficult to free from it.

The process seems to be that the food, or
other foreign matter deposited, undergoes a fer-
mentation and softens the enamel. The softened portion is soon removed, and another surface undergoes a like change, until the substance
of the tooth is laid bare, when the process becomes more rapid, both from the material being
more readily acted upon, and a larger quantity of
the agent being at work.

When decay is discovered in a tooth, immediate steps should be taken to have it remedied.

The remedy consists in removing all the affected part carefully and thoroughly ; and next,
protecting the interior of the tooth thus exposed
from further collection of offensive matter. If
the decay is superficial, it may be filed away ; if
too deep for this, it must be gouged or drilled
out, and to prevent food from collecting in the
cavity, this must be filled up with some substance that will not corrode.

Except near the front of the mouth it is

impossible for a person to inspect many places where decay is very apt to commence.

It is, then, absolutely necessary for the proper preservation of the teeth, that a dentist should be consulted, not only when necessity for his services is made apparent by suffering and inconvenience, but periodically, at intervals not greater than three months; and with those having soft teeth or teeth liable to speedy decay, at even much shorter intervals.

In concluding my remarks on the teeth, I would say that the tooth-pick is an instrument scarcely, if any, less important than the tooth-brush; for it is very desirable that after each meal, as many as possible of the pieces of food which remain between the teeth should be removed.

It should be of such material, and so used, as not to scratch the teeth or injure the gums. Quill, wood, or ivory are all good to make them of, though wood has more of the desirable qualities than the others. Metal should never be used.

As early an opportunity as practicable should

be sought after each meal for picking the teeth. In doing it, take care not to irritate the gums; and having done it, rinse the mouth thoroughly with cold water.

THE NAILS.

The nails grow in two ways—by a deposit from the fine folds of the skin beneath, gradually increasing in thickness; and also by another at the root, which pushes the whole nail forward.

This interesting yet delicate method of forming the nail is very liable to disturbance, and more so by appreciable causes, accidents and the result of carelessness, than by any proneness of Nature to intermit the regular performance of her work.

Blows often interrupt the formation of the nail, destroying the vitality of the cells on the under surface, and thus detaching the nail partially, or even entirely, from the true skin.

This requires the production of an entirely new nail, which, unless the violence has been sufficient to materially impair the nail-making power of the fine folds above described, is a precise reproduction of the old one.

On our feet, the nails are mostly affected by our carelessness in suffering the shoes to press upon them and impede their growth.

In some instances, the growth in length is impeded, and, the formation of nail still going on, it is forced back upon itself, and thickened sometimes to an incredible degree. At other times, pressure on the surface thins and spreads the nail, forcing it into the flesh, or even suppresses entirely its formation, leaving the toe unsupplied with the protection Nature intended for it.

For the preservation of the nails, careful attention is necessary; always keep them from growing too long, by trimming neatly from time to time; keep them from collections of dirt under the free edge, by using a nail-brush or a piece of soft wood;—never use a pen-knife or any sharp pointed instrument. Leave the edge of scarf-skin, near the root, uncut, but push it back, if necessary, with any smooth instrument adapted for the purpose.

I do not think any but a temporary advantage is gained by scraping the nails. At the same time the risk is run of damaging the fine structure on which the excellence of the nail depends.

I need scarcely add here that the habit which some children have of biting the nails should be stopped without delay, as it invariably, if continued for any length of time, permanently deforms them. I have met many ladies who would have been deeply thankful had their parents taken efficient means to break them of a habit which has entailed upon them, thin flattened and distorted nails, and stumpy finger-ends.

Dipping the finger ends into some bitter tincture will generally prevent children from putting them to the mouth, but if this fails, as it sometimes will, each finger end should be encased in a stall, until the propensity is eradicated.

THE FEET.

Upon no part of our persons have the effects of a faulty fashion of dress more strongly impressed themselves than upon the feet, and this so generally that no standard, probably, could be found amongst us, with which we could make such comparisons as would demonstrate the full truth and force of this assertion.

I well remember the first foot I ever saw which had attained to adult age untrammeled by the deforming and stunting influence of a shoe. As much as my knowledge of physiology had prepared me to make, as I thought, ample allowances for the effects of compressed and distorted bones—for displaced tendons and for blighted muscles—I was, nevertheless, surprised greatly at the contrast between the angular and attenuated members that had been encased from childhood in shoes, and the foot to which an Arab sandal had allowed every development that Nature intended.

Full, rounded and even plump in its general form, it yet had great expression in the markings of muscles, well brought out by habitual use. The arch, though not supported, as ours is, by the shoe, still retained an undiminished curve, and gave another proof of the falsity of our notions that Nature ever needs some help of art in retaining her grace of form.

Each toe, regular in its arrangement, and symmetrical in its shape, was tipped with a nail as seemly as that of a finger, and possessed an independence of play and readiness of action, difficult even to be conceived of by those with whom these members have ceased to be active ones, and who, in many instances, only realize their existence by the painfulness of the ex-crescences with which they are furnished.

And why should not the foot have this excellence of form, this elegance of shape? And why should it be restricted in that grace, in that fullness of purpose, for which it was so admirably devised?

Of bones, twenty-six enter into its construction, bound together by more than seventy ligaments. To them are attached the tendons of twelve large muscles, which, though situated upon the leg, by means of multiplied pulleys impress their action even upon the toes ; while twenty more muscles, with various offices, are to be found in the foot itself.

The heel, receiving first the weight of the person in walking, is provided with an elastic cushion to protect it, and to save the rest of the frame from the jar that a less yielding support would give it at every step.

Beneath the arch, this cushion, not so necessary to resist direct pressure, is replaced by a powerful ligament to bind the extremities of the arch together, and to thus·secure firmness to the support when, in the further act of progression, the heel is raised from the ground.

THE SHOES WE WEAR.

There are many faults, to greater or less extent, with all shoes, unless exceptional ones, now worn ; they are too small in length and breadth ; the toe on the inner side is so rounded as to leave no room for the great toe, which has to be bent outwards to suit ; while, in a similar rounding on the outer side, though to a greater degree, the existence of the little toe is entirely ignored, and it has to find a place where it best can—generally under the one next it.

The result of these faults are, from the shoe being too small, the foot is cramped, the proper play and consequently development of all its parts prevented, and the general effects produced above rehearsed.

When the shoe binds on the instep, a very painful little tumor is gradually formed at the most restricted point, often requiring to be cut out, and sometimes implicating, in the inflammation apt to accompany it, the tendon passing alongside of it—that of the muscle which extends the toes.

When too large, the consequences are not so bad ; but the foot is liable, from too great freedom of motion—from being alternately pressed forward into the shoe, and partially lifted out of it again—to chafe, and corns are thus as readily produced as with shoes too tight.

When the shoe is too short, the nails are pushed against their roots, painfully irritating them, and in time producing a thickening and distortion of the former. This, if long continued, can not readily be cured, but remains a source of perpetual annoyance.

When, from fault of shape, the great toe is

thrust outwards, as I have before mentioned, a strain is kept up continually upon its joint with the foot—the ligament soon yields, and an angle is formed.

This, in its projection, receives an undue share of the pressure of the shoe. The least evil that follows is a large bunion—which is a source of never-ceasing annoyance, and one requiring continual care to keep it within the bounds of ordinary endurance.

If it takes on, which it is likely to do, inflammatory action, the joint immediately in contact with it, and already stretched partially open, exposing its delicate internal structure, generally shares in the inflammation, and the trouble becomes a very serious one.

The flesh on each side the nail, which ought not to be raised any more than that on the thumb, is pushed up, so as to entirely imbed each edge, particularly the inner one.

The hard substance pressing into the flesh produces inflammation, frequently of a most tedious and troublesome kind, requiring sometimes that the nail should be torn out, in order to remove the exciting cause, and permit the re-establishment of a healthy action.

In several instances, I have seen the second toe forced up, so as to have to lie upon the edge of the great toe, and that of the third. When this continues for any length of time, it is a tedious and difficult thing to remedy. It is strange that at the first warning it should not be prevented.

Though having the shoe properly made is a preventive against the damage to the foot above described, and though it would be the first step in an effort to remedy such damage, the effects last beyond the cause ; and I therefore offer directions for removing them, or, at least, lessening the annoyance attending them.

CORNS.

When the shoe binds or chafes, a callosity is created on the irritated part. If the warning is taken, the corn may be prevented, and the part will return to its natural condition. But, unfortunately, at this stage it excites little attention. Even when the pain commences, it is generally felt at first only during the day-time, when some extra demand has been made upon the feet, but at night it is easier, and the prospective sufferer is sleepy, the thing is forgotten or disregarded, and so time passes until a thoroughbred corn is established.

Even now much might be done to restore the part to its former state, but seldom is anything rational attempted. A few household remedies, the excellence of which seems generally to consist in their antiquity and mysteriousness, are used, and if they fail the case is looked upon as hopeless. In despair, a doctor is applied to ; but often, long before this is done, the case is beyond his reach.

The Treatment of Corns.—The shoe first being properly fitted, if the corn has just commenced, presents, in fact, only a callosity or thickening of the scarf-skin—it will often not be necessary to do more than to wrap the toe, if the corn is on its outer side, with a soft linen rag well smeared with sweet mutton or beef tallow, doing this faithfully at every morning's toilet.

If it is between the toes, it will suffice to interpose between the corn and the opposing surface a little cotton wool, or a piece of soft moose-leather. This is very simple, but it will prove perfectly effectual, if properly and regularly attended to.

If the affection has gone beyond this, and a regular corn is formed, sensitive at the base, we have to proceed further.

Corns that form on the outside of the little toe, or on the top of the others, are, for the most part, hard and projecting, and until an advanced stage, are not remarkably sensitive.

Those situated between the toes do not project much, but press backwards into the true skin, producing much more rapidly and effectually than the others a disorganization of its delicate structures, and soon affecting the tissues beneath, as above mentioned. In treating corns of either of these kinds, we must commence by removing the scarf-skin. In the soft ones this can readily be done; the hard ones, to facilitate it, should be soaked in warm water; or, what is better, poulticed until they are perfectly softened.

The best instrument for assisting in our endeavors is a pair of scissors with one sharp-pointed blade ; at least this is decidedly the best and less likely than any other to do harm in hands unpractised in surgery. The sharp point should be pushed in flat-wise carefully at one side of the corn, and be carried across to the other.

The sensation of the patient will advise as to how deeply this can be done. When carried across, the blades should be closed, and thus the thickness of epidermis is cut through, leaving a sharp edge on each side the cut. These sharp edges can be readily seized by the thumb and finger nails ; and by these means each half can, if slowly and carefully done, be peeled off from the corn, which should then be covered with soft kid or buck-skin, smeared with mutton tallow.

To guard the tender surface from pressure, a

wad of cotton wool may be placed over it, or, what is better, a piece of soft moose-skin, having a piece cut out of it a little larger than the surface of the corn. The pressure of the shoe, or next toe, it will be seen, will be entirely removed by this from the affected part, and borne by that around.

BUNIONS.

The first step towards the formation of a bunion is wearing a shoe which will bend the great toe outwards, so as to make an angle at its joint with the foot. This angle, receiving not only the continual pressure of a too narrow shoe, but an increased one every time the foot is thrust forward into the shoe, becomes irritated, and something like an incipient corn, only on a more extended scale, is formed.

The treament of bunions may be readily deduced from the directions given about the care and cure of corns.

Happy is she—for women, owing to the greater narrowness of their shoes, in proportion, across the roots of the toes, are more prone to bunions than men—who does not put off such treatment until too late.

Tender Feet.—Many persons, particularly elderly ones, have feet habitually disposed to become chafed and irritated upon very slight cause.

This tendency may be entirely and permanently removed, and the general health and strength of the members greatly increased by the application of the Danish Cure.

Manipulation will wholesomely stimulate the skin and nerves, and freshen the circulation in the whole extremity, making it much less liable to take on diseased action.

CARE OF THE FEET.

The feet should be washed daily and wiped carefully, particularly between the toes, where the scarf-skin is apt to collect.

The nails should be neatly trimmed with the scissors, but not too often or too closely.

As to hosiery—putting aside, just now, the consideration of the material, the seams should not be prominent ; a frequent fault in children's socks, and the hosiery should fit well, not contracting the toes nor leaving loose folds to press the foot.

Children claim particular care for their feet, as much of the mischief from which we suffer in after-life is prepared for us before we are able to take care of ourselves.

At this moment I have the care of a lady suffering from an inverted toe-nail, surmounting a distorted toe, which for ten years she has been trying ineffectully to combat with loose shoes. The toe was bent before she took care of herself, and she has had to carry through life, thus far, the effects of carelessness or ignorance in her parents.

Children are but little apt to complain of any annoyance to their feet until they can endure it no longer, and much of the trouble from which the feet suffer does not at first give warning by pain.

Their shoes should be very carefully looked to, and be made broad and of soft material.

The leather may be strong, but it ought to be particularly soft.

Children should be supplied with but one, or, at most, two pairs of shoes at a time. They often have several, which are used until worn out, the parent forgetting that while the child's foot is growing, the shoes are not. Inattention and thoughtlessness on this one point I conceive to be a prolific source of the deformities of the feet.

On the other hand, persons who have attained their growth will find it advantageous to have a large number of shoes—at least three or four pairs—for ordinary use. This will do away with the necessity of putting on a wet pair, and will give opportunity of having the shoes properly sunned and aired.

Few persons are aware of the extent to which the impression of cold upon the feet is felt by the rest of the system ; and I fear it will be difficult, without enlarging upon the reasons for this more than we can do here, to make the reader fully appreciate it.

I have frequently traced an attack of piles, and many different diseases of the spine and womb, for which the patient was wholly at a loss to account, immediately to walking on a cold ground with shoes too thin.

It should be remembered that the lower branches of all the important truncal organs extend directly to, and end in, the feet. There is the most intimate relation and sympathy existing between the lower extremities and the abdominal and pelvic organs. Therefore, when cold comes in contact with these extremities, the effect is instantaneously felt throughout the entire nervous system.

Inflammation of the bowels, diarrhœa and dysentery, frequently result from exposure of the legs and feet in children, and suppression of the menses and disease of the womb and ovaries, in young ladies.

I am convinced, too, from repeated observations, that the periodical suffering of women is often due to the same cause, not only directly, but indirectly also.

Of graver diseases—those of the chest, for instance—I deem it unnecessary to say anything ; for, by the time they have made a good lodgment in the system, the individual has had her fears excited, and becomes generally careful enough, though possibly too late in her care ; but I am anxious to warn the reader against the above-mentioned sly aggressions upon the health, that come without warning, and in the guise of a slight local affection, and that often effect irremediable harm before they are recognized as at all important.

PART VI.

CHILDREN.

HINTS TO PARENTS.

A KNOWLEDGE of the causes of infantile diseases, and the mortality among children, is more important to women, than information upon any other subject.

When we pause for a moment to reflect upon the many painful and dangerous maladies, to the attacks of which children, from the earliest period of their existence are liable, and by which so large a proportion of them are annually destroyed; and when we consider, also, that in the majority of cases these attacks might easily be avoided, by a proper attention to those external agents, to the influence of which the infant is subjected from the moment of its birth, and which, while they are essential to its existence, become, when counteracted or mismanaged, the cause of nearly all its infirmities and diseases; the doctor does not fulfil his duty, when he neglects to point out and urge the administration of the means by which the occurrence of these diseases may be prevented.

I maintain that it is easy, when in possession of the requisite knowledge, by proper attention, to avoid in a majority of cases the attacks of diseases, which cause so much suffering and so many deaths among children.

Then, is it not clearly the duty of every parent, and all who expect to have the care over children, to spare no efforts to obtain the knowledge which is so requisite for the welfare of the helpless and innocent little ones committed to their charge?

Yet how many parents are so thoughtless and reckless as to the welfare, suffering, and even lives of their children, as to neglect spending the few hours in reading which are required, to obtain the knowledge indispensably requisite for the safety of their children; or, who perhaps think they cannot spare the money to obtain suitable books from which the required information may be derived.

They can pay doctors, and spend nights in nursing, and see their children suffer and die, but not a dollar, nor an hour, are they willing to spare for such information as will enable them to preserve the health and lives of their little ones.

It is all important for young persons who intend to become parents, if they wish to transmit healthy organizations to their children, so to live as to preserve their own organizations in a vigorous and healthy condition; for if they fail, or neglect to do this, their children must inevitably suffer from their folly.

One of the chief causes of the fearful mortality among children is to be found in their inheriting delicate organizations from their parents, which are at birth predisposed to disease, and sometimes already diseased.

Parents who possess delicate constitutions cannot transmit substantial organizations to their children, but they may, by proper care and attention, do much toward giving their children even better organizations than they possess; or by negligence and abuse, they may, by exhausting their own vitality, and deforming their persons, transmit delicacy, deformity and disease to their offspring.

The habit, which many ladies have, of compressing, during pregnancy, the waist, and even the abdomen, by corsets and dresses, is a frequent cause of miscarriage, or abortion; and, when it fails to produce this result, it may cause club-feet, distorted spine, contracted stomach, and other deformities of the child; not that I suppose every case of such deformity, at birth, is caused in this way, but the danger of such a result is so great, that mothers who desire well-formed children may well *beware* how they voluntarily produce the least compression of the waist or abdomen during pregnancy, for a single hour.

A loose dress, fresh air, nourishing food, regular exercise, and cheerful amusements, are all important during pregnancy.

These conditions are necessary to give health and vigor to the mother, without which it is impossible for her child to receive a substantial and healthy organization, which will, with any certainty, survive the days of childhood.

MATERNITY.

During pregnancy women should be more than usually solicitous to keep themselves in sound health, inasmuch as not only their *own* well-being but that of their *offspring* is now involved.

Especially, since the mother's state of mind, at this time, is tolerably certain to be reflected in the child's temperament, should she take care to keep herself calm, cheerful, hopeful ; not filled with terror of the "evil to come," but rather taking it for granted that child-bearing, being a normal, universal function of woman, she may reasonably expect a safe and comfortable deliverance.

So doing, she may also reasonably expect to have a quiet, happy, cooing baby, instead of a nervous, peevish, crying one.

If, furthermore, she wishes the coming man or woman to be of that healthy, symmetrical, well-balanced type, which is described as " a sound mind in a sound body," let her keep her intellectual as well as physical faculties in a state of healthy activity, yet carefully avoiding any temptation to overwork.

Let her read the best books, see the best pictures, converse with the best people, pursue the most elevating studies that come in her way ; in short, lead the broadest, freest, most rational life possible. Especially let her determine that she *will not* be "careful and troubled about many things," probably very small things at that ; things not to be put for one moment into competition with her own and her child's welfare.

Let her shirk her cares rather than be burdened by them ; a little temporary confusion in the household is but a small price to pay for an easy confinement and a rapid recovery.

Gentle exercise should be taken as usual, but with greater watchfulness against over-fatigue.

Jumping, falling, lifting, stooping over, running up and down stairs (go slowly, if you *must* go), reaching far off or high up, standing long with the arms elevated over the head—in short, whatever tends to jar or strain any part of the body, should be carefully avoided.

During the first three months of pregnancy, much good may be done and much suffering prevented by appropriate manipulation.

It will strengthen the organs for their extra work, and greatly assist in keeping the blood in healthy circulation. During the eighth month, manipulation over the spine and ovaries will be found very beneficial.

If, in the habit of taking a cold bath, it will be advisable to substitute a lukewarm bath of salt water, every night, during pregnancy.

Heavy shoes, and heavy skirts, and all uncomfortably weighty clothing, should be discarded during this period.

I would also advise the wearing of a long, easy corset, to support the back and ovaries, but care should be taken to avoid all compression of the body. Plenty of room is needed for natural expansion.

CARE OF VERY YOUNG CHILDREN.

It requires great care to preserve the child, after birth, from suffering, and even from great injury.

Its eyes are unaccustomed to the light, and not able to bear a strong light with impunity ; if light is admitted too freely, inflammation and blindness may ensue.

The light should be excluded from the room at first, but after the first day it should be admitted, and daily increased, until the full light of day can be borne.

The surface of the body and the air passages are unaccustomed to the air, and if great pains is not taken to keep the room warm, especially during the first few washings, cold in the head, or even inflammation of the bronchia, and of the lungs, are liable to result.

In Denmark, women always bathe their new-born infants in milk ; this is far preferable to hot water, and obviates the tendency of contracting colds—usually presented after a warm bath.

It should also be remembered that the child's stomach is unaccustomed to food. Previous to birth it has derived its nourishment directly from the mother, without taxing its digestive organs to any considerable extent, if at all. Now it is to be nourished by the means of food taken into the stomach.

The first nourishment that the child should receive is a small quantity of sugar and water, after this, milk may be given.

The child should not be nursed by its mother until the third day. By that time the breast will contain the proper substantial nourishment required for the maintenance of the child. The child will not suffer from its not being allowed to nurse during the first two or three days, if proper care be taken.

Frequently the child is fed with improper substances, and made sick before it is a day old.

Directly after birth the mother should be given a dose of castor oil; this will open the bowels and produce an easy passage. I do not approve of giving any form of laxitive medicine to new-born infants, the nourishing substance found in the mother's breast—when the infant commences nursing—will be found sufficient for all present emergencies.

It is not uncommon for the skin of the infant to become yellow or jaundiced, within a few days after birth. When this occurs the nurse should give it saffron tea. The yellowness will then generally disappear immediately without further treatment.

The infant requires proper nourishment at regular intervals, but does not require the strong medicines and cathartics which physicians generally prescribe for it. Its organization is too delicate to justify parents and nurses in allowing the administration of these poisons at the hands of doctors.

Dr. John Ellis says: "I am satisfied that many children lose their lives from this domestic drugging; and not a few who are not destroyed are thus rendered feeble and delicate during life.

If parents desire to have crying children, let them commence the use of anodynes and cordials, especially such as contain opium, and they will soon have this kind of music to their hearts' content, for these remedies palliate, for the time, but keep up a disposition to the same trouble for which they are given, and soon add innumerable aches and pains by their own poisonous action, and the babe soon comes to cry for its accustomed dose, and suffer as intensely when it is withheld as the most confirmed opium eater of adult life."

" By the use of such poisons, the various functions of the body are rendered torpid, and the organism partially paralyzed, so that a healthy development is prevented."

" These so-called remedies act specifically upon the brain, impairing its function, and giving rise to various nervous diseases ; and even comparative mental imbecility is sometimes undoubtedly caused by their use."

" If a young child cries excessively, or seems ill, we have good evidence that the laws of its organization are being violated in some direction or other ; and instead of palliating the suffering by an anodyne, we should seek out and remove the cause of the evil."

" The point of a pin may be irritating the skin, or the band may be pinned too tight around the body. I have in more than one instance been called to see children suffering from this latter cause, and have seen all suffering cease the moment the bandage was unpinned. It should never be pinned tightly round the body, but loosely."

" The child may be too hot or too cold, or it may be suffering from improper nourishment."

NURSING.

It is as important to the infant as to the adult, that regularity should be observed in receiving its nourishment.

The comfort and happiness, as well as health, of both mother and child, depend very much upon the cultivation of regular habits ; hence, this subject is worthy of attention. Some sacrifices may be required on the part of the mother, in order to establish such habits as are for the child's best good.

Nursing requires to be conducted with a certain method. It must take place at intervals as well regulated as possible ; the caprices which manifest themselves thus early must be wisely resisted, and bad habits must be avoided ; and when the mother is certain that her child has all which he needs, that he has nursed sufficiently, and that he does not suffer, she must know how to divert his attention, and even be able to bear his cries without yielding to new importunities.

It is not necessary to lay down any fixed rule as to how often a new-born child should nurse ; yet it should not be permitted to nurse too frequently, and the interval should be somewhat regular.

Perhaps, at intervals of from two to three hours during the day, and from three to five hours during the night, would be the average, as to frequency, best adapted to the wants of children until the age of three or four months.

The child should never be allowed, night or

day, to remain at the breast continually, nor should it ever be given the breast simply to quiet its crying, for if this system be pursued much inconvenience will result ; for one or two things must happen.

First—If the child does not cry from absolute pain, a bad habit will be generated ; for the child will cry for the mere gratification of being nursed. This will not only create a great deal of trouble, but will be highly injurious to the stomach itself by occasioning it to be overloaded, and thus producing vomiting, purging, or colic.

Secondly—If the child cries from actual suffering, the food may not do any possible good, or it may much increase the evil by its being given at an improper or unnecessary time.

If an adult takes even a small quantity of food often, say every two or three hours, an unnatural craving soon results, and the digestive organs soon become deranged ; pains in the stomach, flatulence, dyspepsia, etc., ensue. With how much more certainty must the delicate organs of the child be deranged by too frequent nursing or feeding.

The infant may take liquid food more frequently than an adult can solid food, without injury; but its stomach must have seasons of rest, or disease will result, as surely, as in the case of the adult.

Some writers recommend nursing children, even young infants, but three times a day, and they tell us they thrive well when thus nursed. That this is much better than it is to nurse them every hour or two I do not question, still, experience has shown that they may be nursed more frequently than this without harm, say once in three or four hours, during the day, after they are three months old.

It is not only important, but indispensable to the health of the mother, that her sleep be regular, consequently, it is very important that the child should be got into the habit of sleeping at night, without waking more than once or twice at most.

It is neither necessary, nor desirable, that the youngest child should nurse more than once or twice during the eight or nine hours the mother requires for sleep; and, after a few weeks, if nursed at the hour for retiring, it is quite as well for it to sleep until morning; or, at most, not nurse more than once during the night.

If the mother can have her regular rest, she will be much more certain to have a good supply of nourishment, and of a good quality, for her child, than she will if she is disturbed several times during the night.

There are many circumstances which may render nursing by the mother impossible, or not expedient. It sometimes happens, that owing to one cause or another, the nipples are sunken in to such an extent as to render it impossible even to draw them out, so as to enable the infant to nurse. The structure of the breasts may have been so far destroyed by abscesses or disease as to destroy their capacity to furnish nourishment.

These, and various other conditions may render it altogether impossible for the mother to nurse her own child.

Then there are many cases where it is not expedient for the mother to nurse her babe, on her own account, even though the child may thrive.

Some mothers, especially in cities, have a free flow of milk, but are excessively exhausted to the extent of endangering life by nursing.

Unless the mother is sufficiently strong and healthy, and suffering from no serious acute disease, I would advise the employing of a wet nurse, in which case, the nurse should be examined, and her milk analyzed, by a competent physician. Neglect of this precaution is often the occasion of great weakness and suffering to the child.

As soon as the nurse enters upon her duties, have her take a teaspoonful of powdered Turkish Rhubarb, to act slightly upon the child's bowels, which it will do quite as effectually, and much more safely, than if administered by the mouth. This should be repeated twice, at intervals of three days; after that, once a month, as long as the child continues to nurse.

If artificial food is required any time during the first eight days, let it be made of equal parts of milk and warm water, adding a tablespoonful of sugar to the pint. Later on, oatmeal gruel may be used, made as follows : Stir two tablespoonfuls of oatmeal into half a pint of water; boil well; strain; and when cool, add sugar and half a pint of fresh milk. If it is desired to make it still more strengthening, stir in a well-beaten egg.

This will be found most nourishing and fattening food for babies. It can also be taken from the nursing bottle.

Panada, made by mixing together bread, water, sugar, and a very little butter, may also be used. Crackers, and anything containing soda should be avoided.

Any food of which boiled milk is a part will produce constipation. It may sometimes be used to advantage in diarrhœa.

An excellent remedy, which is quite harmless for diarrhœa in infants, is the following, which has frequently proved beneficial, where other remedies have failed : Ten drops of paregoric in boiled milk ; repeat the dose after every two or three discharges until a cure is effected. This may

be given to children one month old and upwards :
at two months, give fifteen drops; and increase
in about the same ratio, for older children.

I would here advise all nurses and mothers,
who are in the habit of carrying children on
one arm mainly, to discontinue this most injurious
practice ; the constant weight on one side throws
the body from its true axis, and is a fruitful
source of curvature of the spine.

The child should be carried as much on one
arm as on the other.

FOOD FOR CHILDREN.

Until children are at least one year of age,
the principal articles of food should consist of
bread and milk—milk boiled with rice and sweet-
ened moderately—plain rice pudding,—roasted
potatoes,—plain puddings of tapioca, arrow-root
or sago,—soft boiled eggs, and simple meat
broths with crumbs of bread or cracker.

I would not advise giving children meat until
they are at least three or four years of age, and,
as a ,general rule, it is better during childhood

and youth to discourage, rather than encourage, the inclination to eat meat, if the young person is strong and healthy without it.

Children should never be allowed a great variety of food at the same meal, nor any which contains the least particle of pepper, or any other spice or condiment, except a moderate quantity of sugar or salt.

Our cooks in this country are the most terrible enemies our children have to encounter, and when we look at the food, of which the children of many thoughtless parents are permitted to eat, it is not surprising that so many die, or grow up poor, puny dyspeptics.

They are often permitted to live almost entirely on articles and substances which should never enter the stomach of a child.

A correspondent of a prominent daily paper says : " While visiting a school in Montreal, I asked the teacher if there were any American children there. She said there were, and she could tell them by their pale faces, bright eyes and nervousness. They learned quicker, but lost so many days during the term from sickness that they did not get along as fast as those who were able to be present constantly. I also took occasion to examine their luncheon baskets, and found the American fare to be a piece of mince pie, the same of pound cake, two doughnuts, a pickle, and a cold sausage ; while the English, Irish and Scotch children had either two days' old bread and butter, or bread and apple, with nothing else."

Butter may be used with moderation when cold, but never in the form of rich gravies.

Plain custard and bread pudding, moderately used, are not objectionable, and sweet, ripe fruits may be used with moderation by children.

Oatmeal and milk should always be a staple article of diet ; it is good both for body and brain, and is very productive in making bone, blood and muscle.

Good rich milk and pure water are the only safe, healthful drinks for children ; the only ones likely to build up a sound vigorous constitution.

The importance of physical development, in the case of infants and young children, cannot be too thoroughly impressed upon the minds of parents and nurses, and a few specific suggestions in regard to their application may not be out of order.

During the first two or three months after birth, the child should be handled but little, and should never be placed in the erect or sitting posture ; nor jolted, nor tossed up and down, for this reason : the bones are soft and pliable, the joints are imperfectly developed, and the muscles are small and feeble, and such violent measures may do great injury to its delicate structure, and cause serious disease or deformity.

It should be permitted to lie quietly in its bed or cot, or carried in the arms in the horizontal position, or allowed to ride in the same position in a small carriage.

ESSENTIAL PRECAUTIONS.

I do not advise rocking, as it is injurious, and may cause unpleasant nervous symptoms, and even diseases of the brain and spine, consequently it should be avoided.

Accustoming children to go to sleep in the arms, or on the lap of the nurse or mother, is injurious to the health of the child, by its being confined in an uncomfortable position, rendered hot by the heat of the body and preventing sound sleep.

Children, especially delicate ones, should always be required to go to sleep in their own bed, placed there while awake and required to lie till sleep comes. This soon becomes a habit; it is better for the child, and saves the mother from an immense amount of drudgery as well as loss of sleep and exposure during the night.

After the first two months the child should be allowed to lie on the bed or on a soft cushion spread upon the floor, and amuse itself and use its limbs freely, which is far better than for it to be held in the arms of a nurse; also there is less . danger of deformity.

Children should not be encouraged nor allowed to sit up too soon, for curvature of the

spine may result. Nor should an attempt be
made to induce it to stand on the feet or walk
too soon, as crooked legs frequently result from
such a course.

Until the child is able to walk it should be
carried into the open air and light frequently,
and spend as much time as practicable out of
doors.

Daily as I witness the delicate, thin, pale-
faced little children who are confined most of
their time in the parlors, sitting-rooms, and nur-
series of the wealthy, and in fact, of all who are
above want, in the goodly city where I reside,
my heart sinks within me at the sad sight of
innocent children perishing for the want of
the necessaries of life—air, light, and out-door
exercise.

Notwithstanding the fearful mortality among
the young children of the wealthy and comfortable livers in every city throughout our land, and
the fact that a majority of those who do not die
young, grow up delicate, nervous, sickly and
worthless; still no systematic effort is made, even

by parents, to rescue these little ones from suffering and an untimely grave.

The children of the poor show by their very looks that they fare better as to food, air, light and exercise, than the children of the rich, except in rare instances of actual starvation.

At best, the air in our cities, even the outdoor air, is not of the purest quality, and the sun's light is dim ; therefore I would not have the child at the age of which we are considering, deprived one moment of their influences during the day, except when at meals.

FROM SIX TO SIXTEEN.

Simplicity and regularity of life are the necessary constituents of a healthy childhood ; the only firm foundation stone upon which a satisfactory superstructure can be reared.

As a rule, American parents forget this truth. At the very time when the " curled darling " of the British or Continental aristocracy is made to lead a quiet, simple, regular life in the nursery and school-room—dining early on two or three plain dishes, walking and exercising several hours daily in the open air, and retiring at nine o'clock—the American child is indulged in late hours, late suppers, indigestible food, and exciting amusements, and secluded from the fresh air, in utter disregard of every law of health.

The consequence is seen in pale, nervous, sickly, irritable, children; who cannot do otherwise than to grow up into pale, nervous, sickly, over-worked, and early worn-out adults.

For obvious reasons, my remarks will apply mainly to girls. As I have before stated, boys early take the matter of exercise, at least, into their own hands; and sooner cease to be the objects of motherly anxiety, as regards their physical training.

At six years of age, children may be allowed almost all kinds of food, if plainly cooked and judiciously proportioned. Ripe fruit is always excellent, if not eaten in excess. Tea and coffee should be withheld until the system is fully developed : milk should be used instead.

Until sixteen years of age, children should

retire at nine o'clock. They should not attend evening parties, nor be subjected to any similarly unhealthy excitement.

Throughout this volume I have insisted upon exercise, as indispensable to sound health ; yet much injury is done to girls by so-called health exercises.

Jumping-the-rope, skating, and gymnastic exercises, the *manner* and movements of which have not been examined and recommended by a competent physician, may be set down generally as doing more harm than good.

During my practice, I have had numerous cases of weakness, contractions, and rupture, caused by these exercises alone. The injuries likely to arise from injudicious exercises, have been more fully explained in the previous pages of this work, and more particularly under the headings " The Gymnasium," " Dumb-Bells," etc.

Girls should be carefully taught to sit upright, and not allowed to lean over desks, or sit in bent, cramped positions at their books or work ; for these positions tend to narrow the chest, and predispose to lung diseases.

A few moments should be spent every day in teaching them the art of perfect breathing, by expanding the chest fully, and making the inspirations long and deep as possible.

The time will not only be well spent, but it will be an actual saving in the end, inasmuch as whatever tends to make a child healthy, relieves the mother of many an anxious hour's watch by a sick bed.

The essentials in the clothing of children, are *lightness*, *simplicity*, and *looseness*.

By its being as light as is consistent with due warmth, it will neither encumber the child, nor cause any waste of its powers; in consequence of its simplicity, it will be readily and easily put on, while by its looseness, it will give full room for the growth and regular expansion of the entire frame, and allow freedom of action to all the limbs and muscles; a matter of infinite importance for the securing of health and comfort in after life.

From six years of age upwards, I would recommend girls to wear a simple easy corset—not to lace the figure, but to keep it upright and support the developing organs. It should be made without steels ; substitute two whalebones in the back and one in the front, these bones to be an inch and a half wide and quite stiff. This will furnish support for the spine and other organs, which are so easily injured at this early age..

Girls approaching womanhood—that is to say, from twelve to sixteen years old—should be carefully watched. Over-fatigue, either of body or brain, should be sedulously guarded against ; so also should all nervous excitement.

Food, exercise, study and amusement, should all be wisely regulated in such a manner as to afford the most assistance, and do the least harm, to the rapidly developing system.

The food should be of the most nourishing, strengthening kind, but not stimulating. The exercise should be regular without being violent.

Teachers should be requested not to exact too much in the way of study, at certain times, nor to permit the pupil to sit too long at the desk, or in any one position.

The amusements should be simple and joyous, leaving, so to speak, a good taste behind; not so artificial and exciting as to be followed by a depressing reaction.

Finally, the reasons why such and such precautions, and such a regimen, are necessary, should be calmly and seriously stated to the child; false modesty in this direction is the parent of numerous evils. Give girls to understand in time the peculiarities and necessities of their sex, and remember that " to be forewarned is to be forearmed."

The time of life at which menstruation, or the monthly discharge, occurs, varies according to circumstances. The most influential agents in retarding or hastening the discharge are climate and habits of life.

In warm climates the courses come on as early as from eight to twelve years; in more temperate regions they may be expected at from twelve to sixteen; and as late as from fifteen to twenty in cold countries. In this country the average might be placed at fifteen in the Southern States, and a little later at the North.

A country life and occupations, simple manners and frugal fare, tend to retard the appearance of the courses. On the contrary, an easy life of self-indulgence, stimulating food and drinks, attending balls and children's parties, and the whole hot-bed system of city life, all stimulate the sexual organs into precocious activity, which is followed by a premature old age—"'Neath whose withering touch the lines of beauty fade away."

As soon as girls show any signs of maturing, it will be well to give them, every other night, on going to bed, a teacupful of catnip tea, adding a half-teaspoonful of saffron. It will render needed assistance to the system. At the same time, rub the back and hips well, but avoiding pressure on the ovaries. This will produce a healthy action of the spleen ; also rub the bottom of the feet, to assist the circulation.

During menstruation, it is best not to lie

down and give up to a feeling of languor or discomfort, however strong the inclination to do so. Gentle exercise will greatly assist the discharge and also strengthen the organs.

The discharge should not continue over three days; after that time, regulate it by taking the following :

Mix two tablespoonfuls of ground cinnamon with a pint of water ; add two tablespoonfuls of lemon juice and the outer rind of a lemon ; drink the pint in a day. It will prove an efficient and pleasant regulator.

If there is *much* pain attending menstruation, use a hot sitz bath ; hop tea is better than water alone.

The pain is caused by nervous contraction of the organs, and the bath will relax them in from ten to fifteen minutes. Immediately after the bath, lie down for two or three hours.

If the pain is constant and severe, manipulation will be most servicable. It must be done, however, by a person skilled in the art, as well as thoroughly acquainted with anatomy.

Finally, in concluding this subject, I would

insist on the importance of having young girls informed as to the nature of menstruation, the time of its appearance, etc., etc.

In the absence of such knowledge, attempts have been made to check it by the use of cold water and other dangerous means. And without a knowledge of the nature and uses of this function, some of the most important truths of Nature must be suppressed.

The fact is, there is too much fastidiousness and false delicacy in this age of the world, which should be banished ; and young girls, as soon as they reach the proper age, should be instructed fully in everything pertaining to the preservation of that greatest and most desirable of all earthly blessings—health.

PART VII.

DISEASES PECULIAR TO WOMEN.

THE attention and candid consideration of my readers, as to what I have to say regarding the common affections of the procreative organs, is earnestly desired. It will not do to pass this subject over as too delicate for investigation.

If the subject is delicate, the complex generative organization is also delicate, and a vast amount of human suffering, not only to women themselves, but to posterity, results from a foolish ignorance on the part of many females—old and young—who shut their eyes upon everything calculated to teach them how to preserve the strength and healthfulness of the organs peculiar to their sex.

Our grandmothers were not so much the slaves of pernicious customs and fashions, as those who are in future to become grandmothers, and consequently, many precautions which are necessary to maintain health to-day, were not necessary in their day and generation.

Young unmarried women, and young mothers, have died in all ages of the world ; a large number of whom might have been saved to become grandmothers, had they properly understood and regarded all the laws of life and health.

Uterine diseases are becoming so general, that women entirely exempt from them, are more rarely to be met with than those who are suffering to a greater or less extent with them in some form.

PROLAPSUS UTERI, OR FALLING OF THE WOMB.

As this disease has become so common and general, both with the young and unmarried as well as with others, and as so few dream of the true nature of their difficulty, and of the requisite remedy, or of its necessary application, I will give a succinct description of the malady, leaving out many of the associated symptoms which sometimes accompany, and which have been referred to in the different parts of this work.

Generally, the complaint will come on by degrees. The patient will begin to lose her power of endurance more and more, the back begins to ache before noon, or night, and this may exist in every variety of degree, even to terrible pain, wrangling and twisting, and making the back feel as if it were broken, or pounded.

This is generally in the region of the kidneys, small of the back, or spinal column, and may be distressingly severe in the spine, low down ; the patient will also feel a sense of dragging in the groins, a twisting and wringing, which, in connection with the sense of weight at the bottom of the abdomen, renders the sufferer often so miserable, that she sits down in the midst of her cares, and cries out in anguish and despair.

She moves carefully, and holds herself by the hand at the lower part of the body, to prevent being jarred or jolted. She walks bent over to avoid that dragging in the breast, which is such a constant attendant on this affliction.

The limbs will often have cramps or spas-

17

modic movements, and the spine and hips also attended with severe pain.

Although she may be somewhat smart in the morning, or on certain days, yet the limbs generally will by noon become heavy and clumsy; the patient will feel as though the hips were loose, and that brisk movements would be attended with injury and great displacement of the internal organs.

These, and other symptoms not here mentioned, may, and do, exist in endless varieties of degree; more commonly in moderate and endurable degree, so that the patient can go about attending to her ordinary avocations, but suffering more or less.

This is especially the case with young ladies who are ignorant of the true character of the complaint, and know only how uncomfortable they are, and *not* how much they need beneficial treatment, nor how much they are undermining their constitutions and unfitting themselves for future usefulness.

While on this point, let me say to my dear young lady readers who feel that they are beginning to come under this description, do not deceive and abuse yourselves; you conceal from both *mother* and doctor the facts, because you suppose that such afflictions usually belong to the sex, and that, should you make known your true state, wrong impressions as to your chastity and purity would be entertained.

It is *not* so, my young friends; this malady is not of local origin or perpetuity. It is *not* the least indication, one way or the other, on the point conceived; it is but the result of a relaxation of the muscles and ligaments of the trunk generally, which is as likely to afflict the young and chaste girl as the *old* or married woman.

Then cease to abuse yourselves on this point; fly to relief early, and arrest the stealthy destroyer, with a light, cheerful, and innocent heart. Do not delay till you are *compelled* to act, and thus have rendered the hope of success more dubious.

Frequently this disorder can be traced directly

to a diseased condition of the spine, and perhaps *more* often is the cause thus due traced to this source, than to any other organ.

When the muscles of the spine, abdominal muscles, or those of the womb itself, become weakened, and relaxed from insufficient stimuli, or when a pernicious fashion induces a woman of not very strong muscular organization to compress her waist so as to press down the stomach and bowels below their normal position, the advent of this most distressing disease may very reasonably be looked for.

Child-bearing and too early getting up after confinement, have been mentioned by some writers as being among the causes; but it is my opinion that these things would but seldom result in falling of the womb, if women would leave off their enervating habits, and live so as to give strength and firmness to their muscles.

To suppose that falling of the womb is a necessary result of child-bearing, in itself, is to impugn the wisdom and goodness of the Almighty, and to say that he has imposed a duty on woman which she cannot perform, except at the sacrifice of health and comfort. Can any one believe this?

As I have before stated, the principal cause of this, and many other diseases of the procreative organs, is caused by a relaxation of the muscles.

While speaking of the causes, it may be proper to explain a little more fully *how* relaxation of the muscles of the abdomen causes falling of the womb. This will serve to show the importance of using means to strengthen the relaxation.

When these muscles are firm and strong, any one can see in a moment that they must press the stomach, liver, bowels, and all the contents of the abdomen, upwards and backwards; whereas, if they are relaxed, they will yield to the pressure from within, and allow the organs to push forward and press downward, crowding on the womb.

I have frequently encountered cases of prolapsus of the womb, in my practice, in which there was no unpleasant symptoms whatever.

The displacement had occurred at such an early age that the system had been made gradually to tolerate its unnatural position. But an examination reveals the true state of affairs; and it is generally found, in cases of this kind, that their ill health proceeds, directly or indirectly, from this uterine displacement.

Leucorrhœa generally precedes, and in most cases attends, falling of the womb. Unless relieved or cured, months or years of misery, according to the endurance of the sufferer, are fastened upon her, until consumption, or some other disease in a fatal form, forever relieves her of her physical distress.

In the incipient stages of the disease the exercise of walking is necessary to keep up what is left of the muscular strength; but in advanced stages this exercise is generally too painful to be endured; then daily manipulation of the abdomen should be resorted to.

The natural action of the abdominal muscles, when in health, and all acting in concert, is upward and backward. Consequently, the more healthy and elastic these organs are, the more perfectly will they effect this perpetual elevation and protection of the pelvic viscera.

Judicious pressure with the hands, imitating the action of the muscles, in the region of the spine and abdomen, will do more towards restoring a healthy action, to these muscles, than any other method known to science, or the medical fraternity.

Of course, attention should be given to the observing of a proper regime during treatment. Let her commence taking moderate exercise in a carriage, and increase in activity as the powers of life arise. Let her cultivate the habit of constantly sitting erect, and throwing back her shoulders. Never let her lace her waist at all. Let her rise early and take the air, and to retire early will be of advantage.

By pursuing this course, in conjunction with what has already been mentioned, every patient will be restored from a confinement of even many years to perfect health.

PART VIII.

CARE OF THE SICK.

When sickness enters a family, there is great need of each member giving strict attention to personal cleanliness, and diet, to preserve themselves in a healthful condition, and by thus doing, fortify themselves against disease.

It is also of the greatest importance that the sick-room, from the first, be properly ventilated. This will be beneficial to the afflicted, and highly necessary to keep those well who are compelled to remain a length of time in the sick-room.

It is of vital importance to the sick to have an even temperature in the room. This cannot always be correctly determined, if left to the judgment of attendants, for they may not be the best judges of a right temperature. And some persons require more heat than others, and would be only comfortable in a room which to others would be uncomfortably warm.

And if each of these are at liberty to arrange the fires, to suit their ideas of proper heat, the atmosphere in the sick-room will be anything but regular.

Sometimes it will be distressingly warm for the patient; at another time too cold, which will have a most injurious effect upon the sick.

The friends of the sick, or attendants, who through anxiety and watching, are deprived of sleep, and who are suddenly awakened in the night from sleep to attend in the sick-room, are liable to chilliness. Such are not correct thermometers of the healthful temperature of a sick-room.

In pleasant weather the sick in no case should be deprived of a free supply of fresh air. Their rooms may not always be so constructed as to allow the windows or doors open in their rooms, without the draught coming directly upon them and exposing them to take cold. In such cases windows and doors should be opened in an adjoining room, and thus let the fresh air enter the room occupied by the sick.

Fresh air will prove more beneficial to the sick than medicine, and is far more essential to them than their food. They will do better, and recover sooner, deprived of food, than of fresh air.

Many invalids have been confined weeks and months in close rooms, shutting out the light, and pure invigorating air of heaven, as though air was a deadly enemy, when it was just the medicine they wanted to make them well.

The whole system was debilitated and diseased for want of air, and Nature was sinking under her load of accumulating impurities, in addition to the fashionable poisons administered by physicians, until she was overpowered and broke down in her efforts, and the sick died.

They might have lived had proper treatment been administered. They died victims to their own ignorance, and that of their friends, and the ignorance and deception of physicians who gave them fashionable poisons, and would not allow them pure water to drink, and fresh air to breathe, to invigorate the vital organs, purify the blood, and help Nature in her task in overcoming the bad conditions of the system.

These valuable remedies which Nature has provided, without money and without price, were cast aside and considered not only as worthless, but even as dangerous enemies, while poisons, prescribed by physicians, were in blind confidence taken.

Thousands have died from want of pure water and pure air, who might have lived; and thousands of living invalids, who are a burden to themselves and others, think that their lives *depend* upon taking medicines from doctors.

They are continually guarding themselves against the air, and avoiding the use of water.

If they would become enlightened, and let medicine alone, and accustom themselves to out-door exercise, and to pure air in their houses, summer and winter, they would be comparatively well and happy, instead of dragging out a miserable existence.

It is the duty of attendants and nurses in the sick-room to have a special care of their own health, especially in critical cases of fever and consumption.

One person should not be kept closely confined to the sick-room. It is safer to have two or three to depend upon, who are careful and understanding nurses, and these changing and sharing the care and confinement of the sick-room. Each should have exercise in the open air as often as possible.

This is important to sick-bed attendants, especially if the friends of the sick are among that class who continue to regard air, if admitted into the sick-room, as an enemy, and will not allow the windows raised or the doors opened. The sick and the attendants are in this case compelled to breathe the poisonous atmosphere from day to day, because of the inexcusable ignorance of the friends of the sick.

In very many cases the attendants are ignorant of the wants of the system, and the relation which the breathing of fresh air sustains to health, and the life-destroying influence of inhaling the diseased air of a sick-room.

In this case the life of the sick is endangered, and the attendants themselves are liable to take on disease, and lose health and perhaps life.

If fever enters a family, often more than one have the same fever. This need not be, if the habits of the family are correct. If their diet is as it should be, and they observe habits of cleanliness, and realize the necessity of ventilation, the fever need not extend to another member of the family.

The reason of fever prevailing in families, and exposing the attendants, is because the sick-room is not kept free from poisonous infection by cleanliness and proper ventilation.

The mother, from a sense of duty, has left her family to administer in the sick-room, where pure air was not allowed to enter, and has become sick by inhaling the diseased atmosphere, which affected her whole system. After a period of much suffering, she has died, leaving her children motherless. The sick, who shared the sympathy and

unselfish care of this mother, recovered, but neither the sick, nor the friends of the sick, understood that precious life was sacrificed because of
their ignorance of the relation which pure air
sustains to health.   Neither did they feel responsibility in regard to the stricken flock, left without the tender mother's care.

Mothers sometimes permit their daughters to
take care of the sick in illy ventilated rooms, and,
as a result, have had to nurse them through a
period of sickness.   And because of the mother's anxiety and care for her child, she has been
made sick, and frequently one or both have died,
or been left with broken constitutions, or made
suffering invalids for life.

There is a lamentable catalogue of evils, which
have their origin in the sick-room, from which
pure air is excluded.   All who breathe this poisonous atmosphere violate the laws of their being
and must suffer the penalty.

The sick, as a general thing, are taxed with
too many visitors and callers, who chat with them,
and weary them by introducing different topics

of conversation, when they need quiet and undisturbed rest.

It is a mistaken kindness that leads so many, out of courtesy, to visit the sick. Often have they spent a sleepless, suffering night, after receiving visitors. They have been more or less excited, and the reaction has been too great for their already debilitated energies, and, as the result of these fashionable calls, they have been brought into very dangerous conditions, and lives have been sacrificed for the want of thoughtful prudence.

It is sometimes gratifying to the sick to be visited, and to know that friends have not forgotten them in their affliction. But, although these visits may have been gratifying, in very many instances, these fashionable calls have turned the scale when the invalid was recovering, and the balance has borne down to death.

Those who cannot make themselves useful should be cautious in regard to visiting the sick. If they can do no good, they may do harm. But the sick should not be neglected.

They should have the best of care and the sympathy of friends and relatives.

Much harm has resulted to the sick from the universal custom of having watchers at night.

In critical cases this may be necessary; but it is often the case that more harm is done the sick by this practice than good.

It has been the custom to shut out the air from the sick-room. In addition to this, to have one or two watchers to use up the little vital air which may find its way to the sick-room through the crevices of doors and windows, is taking from them this vitality, and leaving them more debilitated than they would have been had they been left to themselves.

The evil does not end here. Every one watcher will make more or less stir, which disturbs the sick. But where there are two watchers, they often converse together, sometimes aloud, but more frequently in whispered tones, which is far more trying and exciting to the nerves of the sick than talking aloud.

Many suffering, wakeful nights are endured

by the sick because of watchers. If they were left alone, knowing that all were at rest, they could much better compose themselves to sleep, and in the morning they would awake refreshed.

Every breath of vital air in the sick-room is of the greatest value, although many of the sick are very ignorant on this point. They feel very much depressed, and do not know what the matter is. A draught of pure air through their room would have a happy, invigorating influence upon them.

All unnecessary noise and excitement should be avoided in the sick-room, and the whole house should be kept as quiet as possible.

Ignorance, forgetfulness and recklessness, have caused the death of many who might have lived had they received proper care from judicious, thoughtful attendants.

The doors should be opened and shut with great care, and the attendants should be unhurried, calm and self-possessed. The sick-room, if possible, should have a draught of air through

18

it, day and night. The draught should not come directly upon the invalid. While burning fevers are raging there is but little danger of taking cold. But especial care is needed when the crisis comes, and fever is passing away. Then constant watching may be necessary to keep vitality in the system.

At this stage, nothing will prove more beneficial and efficacious, in strengthening and increasing the vitality, than electricity, imparted to the system by manipulation.

It strengthens more surely than any tonic. The feeble patient gets the benefit of exercise without the fatigue. The muscles are made to act, and the blood to circulate freely, without any expenditure of nervous forces.

This treatment tends not only to hasten the patient's return to health, but by quickening the circulation, it strengthens the activity of the blood-vessels, thereby causing the removal of all poisonous and foreign substances from the circulation, and, by so doing, it imparts new life and strength to the entire system.

This treatment applied to women in health, will act as a preventive against disease.

A great amount of suffering might be saved if all would labor to prevent disease, by strictly obeying the laws of health. Strict habits of cleanliness should also be observed.

Many while well, will not take the trouble to keep in a healthy condition. They neglect personal cleanliness, and are not careful to keep their clothing pure. Impurities are constantly and imperceptibly passing from the body, through the pores, and if the surface of the skin is not kept in a healthy condition, the system is burdened with impure matter. And if the garments worn are not frequently cleansed from these impurities, the pores of the skin absorb again the waste matter thrown off.

The impurities of the body, if not allowed to escape, are taken back into the blood, and forced upon the internal organs. Nature, to relieve herself of poisonous impurities, makes an effort to free the system; which effort produces fevers, and what is termed disease. But even then, if those who are afflicted would resort to proper treatment, to assist Nature in her efforts, much suffering would be prevented.

But many instead of doing this, and seeking to remove the poisonous matter from the system, take a more deadly poison into the system to remove a poison already there. It is well known, that physicians frequently prescribe mineral poisons for curing fevers. These poisons, instead of curing fevers, increase the already existing fever, and when fever does not exist they create it.

The evils, resulting from the use of these powerful preparations, have been commented upon at length, under the heading of " Drugs."

If every family realized the beneficial results of thorough cleanliness, they would make special efforts to remove every impurity from their persons, and from their houses—which are frequently at fault, and often found to be the direct cause of what physicians call " malarial " fevers.

THE
"DANISH CURE"
EXPLAINED.

" Without some knowledge of anatomy and physiology, directions for the preservation of health cannot be thoroughly appreciated —symptoms are without meaning, and the use of remedies a blind experiment."

ALTHOUGH this cure is comparatively a new one in this country, it has been recognized as an established and important branch of General and Scientific Anatomy, in Germany and Denmark, since the fifteenth century; and the success achieved by this method of treatment, in chronic diseases, has exceeded that of any other branch of medical science in these countries.

While visiting an institution at Copenhagen, Denmark, my attention was arrested, on seeing this treatment administered to a patient, by one of the practitioners in charge.

On making inquiry as to the nature of the treatment, I was struck with the great advantage this cure possessed over the common method of treatment by drugs.

Continuing my inquiries among the patients, I found there existed with them all a steady progress toward a complete restoration to health.

I found cases of deformity and distortion of *twenty years'* standing, where the patient had received the attendance of the most eminent medical men of Europe, but without avail.

I found cases of double and triple spinal curvature ; where the patient had been compelled to support an iron corset of *fifty pounds weight*, for years, in the vain hope of restoring the spine to its normal condition.

I also found cases of contractions and distortions, hideous to behold ; patients whose limbs, the cords of which were so contracted—from rheumatism and other causes—as to draw the lower limbs up to the head.   Almost all of these patients had been confined to their bed for years, and pronounced incurable by physicians.

On noticing the improvement made from day to day, by these so-styled incurable patients, under this method of treatment, a great desire possessed me to become a practitioner, and assist suffering humanity in getting rid of these unsightly deformities of person—and diseases in general—the majority of which can not be removed by medicinal treatment.

Following my desire, I studied anatomy carefully and thoroughly, in the dissecting room of the Langaard Institute, at Copenhagen, under the tuition of my uncle, Dr. Emile Fresch, Physician to King Christian the Eighth, of Denmark.

Here also, I was instructed in the science of manipulation at a later period.

I would here state that the study of anatomy, in Denmark, is pursued in altogether a different manner from what it is in this country. Here, the knowledge of the human frame is derived *altogether* from the dissecting room—by the dissection of a lifeless body. This knowledge is all very well in locating the different bones, muscles, cords, etc., and tracing their connection with the different organs in the system ; but it does not furnish the necessary information on the most important characteristic of anatomy, namely : the action of the constituent elements of our body, and the influence they possess over other organs, of greater or less importance, in the system.

In Denmark the study of anatomy is conducted in a somewhat different manner. After completing a course of study in the dissecting-room, and becoming familiar with the location of those small parts which constitute the great whole, from studying the anatomy of a lifeless body, the student next enters a department devoted entirely to studying the action of the mechanical parts, while in a *living state.*

Here the subjects are live persons ; and the action of the organs, muscles, cords, etc., are carefully studied under different circumstances ; each in turn is carefully traced, and its power and influence over that part of the system in which it is located—as well as the influence it indirectly possesses in parts of the system over which it has no control—correctly noted.

This information cannot be gained by studying *only* the mechanical parts of a lifeless body; hence, the advantage of the Danish system of studying anatomy will be apparent.

A successful practitioner of the Danish Cure, should continue the study of anatomy, until able to detect instantly, upon examination *by the hands alone*, a displacement, contraction, or abnormal condition of any muscle or cord in the body.

The next requirement is to remove this abnormal condition, and restore the affected part to health.

In order to do this, the practitioner must possess an amount of animal electricity sufficient for all emergencies, and a knowledge of how to impart it to the patient, to successfully employ it.

The reader will readily perceive, that not every one so inclined can become a practitioner of this treatment ; as probably not *one* person in *fifty* possesses an amount of electricity sufficient to withstand the effects of administering treatment to a dozen or two patients daily—(which is about my average practice)—and retain enough electricity to support their own constitutions, and be able to continue the treatment day after day.

On coming to this country, I found this cure entirely unknown, and with me remains the credit of introducing it in America.

The *Swedish Movements*, introduced in this country some years ago, is essentially different in principle, and should not be confounded with the Danish Cure.

The following unsolicited letter, from Dr. J. Rutherford Wooster, of New York City, may be of interest in explaining the requisite qualifications of a successful practitioner.

This letter is only one of many received from eminent men in New York and other cities. But I shall refrain from publishing them, as this treatment needs only to be explained to be appreciated.

New York, Dec. 18—.

The "Danish Cure," introduced by Mme. Wilhelmine D. Schott, of this city, has many points to commend it to favorable consideration. A neat volume recently published by the lady may be taken as a fair exponent of her "modus operandi." But in all operations where personal contact is necessary, the operator should be healthy in body, mild and gentle in disposition and speech ; yet "*suaviter in modo, but fortiter in re,*" are indispensable elements, for a successful practitioner.

This lady is peculiarly blessed with a fine physique and remarkable *magnetic and will power*, to ensure success in this mode of treating disease.

No feeble or defective organism, of body or mind, should attempt to treat disease by manipulation.

Madame Schott is blessed with a full, symmetrical form and a noble, womanly presence ; her manners bland and pleasing, so much so that she secures at once the confidence, love and respect of her patients, which is half the cure.

Having taken occasion to visit the establishment, on several admission seasons, and conversing with those under treatment, I have noticed a marked and steady improvement in all her cases, which are generally of a chronic character. Her book is its own interpreter, setting forth facts which no candid person can gainsay. Too much abstruse philosophy eclipses knowledge to the masses, in these days of advanced civilization.

After a careful perusal of the first edition of " Health Hints to Women," I find nothing to condemn, but much to approve, and most heartily commend it to the attention of the ladies, as tending to the light of a clearer knowledge of themselves and their mission.

J. RUTHERFORD WOOSTER, M. D.

My practice has always been confined to the cure of chronic diseases of women and children— mainly to those who have been "given up" and pronounced "incurable" by physicians. In the treatment of these diseases I have been even more successful than I ever dared anticipate.

The following letter, which, by chance I still have in my possession, was written by Dr. Taylor during the first year of my practice in this country.

WOMEN'S HOSPITAL,
NEW YORK, Dec. 6, 1871.

To Mme. WILHELMINE D. SCHOTT,
Aberdeen Hotel.

DEAR MADAME :—The Lady Managers of this institution join their grateful thanks to those of our lady patients, for your disinterested, humane and invaluable services rendered them recently, in the application of your method of treatment, which has certainly proved very effective.

In view of these facts, we should be glad to make some arrangement whereby your valuable services may be confined exclusively to this institution.   Should this proposition meet with your wishes, we will be pleased to accept any proposal you may choose to make.

Very respectfully yours,

K. R. TAYLOR,

House Surgeon.

The first step in the application of the Danish Cure, is a thorough examination of all the organs — internally and externally — the muscles, cords, tendons, etc., and more particularly the spine and rectum.

The internal organs which require the most rigid examination, are, the neck of the womb, the ovaries, the bladder, the urethra, and the rectum.

Of the above-mentioned organs, the spine is the most fruitful source of disease.

The lower extremity, or point, of the spine is rounded, when a person enjoys good health, and when in poor health, or any disease exists in that organ, it is pointed. By touching the point of the spine, a tingling sensation is at once felt in the head. This point is very susceptible to injury, on account of its being very sensitive, and when hurt or pressed, productive of great pain. At this point of the spine, several cords extend to the neck of the womb ; these cords require a careful examination for the reason that when they are injured, or contracted, displacement of the womb frequently follows. This displacement causes constipation, piles, and other evils which follow in its train.

A careful and thorough examination will disclose the original cause of any disorder, and by removing the cause which produced the disease, the disease can be cured with greater certainty.

The next point to be considered is, how to remove the original cause when traced to its proper source.

If due to any mechanical disarrangement, I

maintain that the removal can be accomplished *more effectually*, *permanently*, and *easily*, by manipulation, than by any other method known to the medical fraternity.

By manipulation, I do not mean merely rubbing, or producing friction, as some are disposed to think ; nor can any person administer this treatment of manipulation, with any degree of success, unless perfectly familiar with the correct location of every muscle and cord in the body.

This is indispensable for the following reasons: should the muscular system be weak and require attention, not only *one* of the muscles, but *all* of them require strengthening.

The cause of muscles becoming weak is due to the fact of other muscles contracting in some part of the muscular system.

The contraction of cords or muscles, in any part of the system, will be followed by a corresponding relaxation of some other muscles or cords—generally those of the spine. Hence, not only the muscles where weakness or contraction exist need strengthening, but all the other muscles as well.

Manipulation of the muscles is performed by gently stretching them with both hands. This produces an elasticity of action which causes them to raise, thereby increasing their power to act. This treatment is applied mainly with the fingers.

When the nervous system requires attention, the finger ends are used to invigorate the nerves; for the reason that electricity is more readily imparted from a person's finger ends than elsewhere.

The nerves should be gently pressed in one direction and another, which tends to increase their strength and vitality.

In administering manipulation to increase the circulation, the hands should be lightly moved over the surface of the blood-vessels—not rubbing them briskly—but using enough force to quicken the circulation. By strengthening the circulation, injurious substances are more easily removed and a healthy action established.

My first step in treating patients, after examination, is to purify the entire system, to remove
the poisonous effects of medicine previously
taken, though it may have been taken into the
system years ago.

This is done by giving a half teaspoonful of
powdered rhubarb, stirred in a half tumblerful of
water, on retiring, during the first three days;
after this time it depends altogether upon the
condition of the patient as to how often it should
be used.

Powdered rhubarb purifies the liver, acts
upon the kidneys, removes all impurities from the
circulation, and will be found very beneficial,
even to persons enjoying good health, who
should use it at least once a month, to keep the
system free from the impurities which are constantly entering the mechanical organs from some
source or other.

There is in the community a very large class
of women who might be called *half-invalids*—
persons who do not possess a satisfactory amount
of health, but who at the same time feel that

19

they are not the proper subjects for medical care.

Such persons feel that they are forewarned of disease, and would gladly attempt to avert it, could they obtain such directions for doing so as would meet the approbation of their reason, or instinctive sense of physiological propriety.

Medical practice takes no cognizance of these cases, or if it does, it is in such a way as often to confirm the subject in serious and prolonged disease.

Aware of this fact, many keep aloof from medical advice of any kind, and insist that suffering in any of the more moderate forms is less a misfortune than the habit of continually gulping drugs for the palliation they afford.

For all persons of this class, it is evident that it is not drugs, but treatment of the kind explained in this volume, that is required.

By this means, the latent powers which some possess are developed into activity and harmony, and they soon rejoice in health, while the neglect or continued misdirection of these, would eventually have degenerated into grave, and perhaps fatal, disease.

Besides these, there are many whose avocations are sedentary, yet such as require the continued and often severe employment of a part of their muscles. This tends to an undue and disproportionate activity of some parts of the body to the detriment of others.

Such avocations constitute in many constitutions a potent cause of ill health ; but the ill effects of them can be easily counteracted by a recourse to such means as are prescribed in this treatise.

Persons suffering from the causes here alluded to, will be enabled to remove fatigue and congestion from the parts of the body that have been abused by too constant exercise, and greatly strengthen the weakened members, by appropriate manipulation.

The following case shows the truth of my views on the philosophy of manipulation, and also that when the body is weak and droops, it is not from weakness of the spine, but of its *muscles*, or a part of them.

It also shows that the way to cure curvature, or inability to walk or stand, is not to fix a leaning post for the patient, nor to put her in screws so that she cannot fall; for, in this way, the muscles are more palsied by doing for them what Nature should do. In the other case, it compresses the muscles and prevents their action.

In these cases the patient straightens, because she *cannot* crook, stands because she *cannot* fall, and the weak muscles, that so greatly need strength, are gaining nothing by exercise and partial support.

Steel or brass jackets, in the main, only tend to perpetuate the evil. They do not strengthen or enervate the muscles, but, on the contrary, are a productive source of paralysis, when coming in contact with them; besides, the patient is apt to depend upon it, and when it is removed she is lost, and droops down again.

But, by manipulation, the weight is gradually removed from the spine, through the lifting up of the body, caused by strengthening the muscles; also, all the muscles of the back are strengthened and made more tense, causing them to pull back the shoulders, thus causing as much weight to rest behind the axis of the body as before it.

The facts of this case are as follows :

Miss H., of Brooklyn, N. Y., a young and beautiful lady, had lost one sister of irritation and distortion of the spine ; she died under the ordinary treatment of brass stays, jackets, severe lacing and pressure.

She herself was verging to the same condition, and had visited a medical institution which gave special attention to these complaints.

She wore a brass corset or jacket, which nearly reached round her ; it covered her whole back. When it was laced on she could remain quite straight by leaning on it, but on removing it she was lost and "gone," as she said.

The constant wearing of this metal corset produced a most injurious effect upon the muscles of the back, by the severe pressure upon them. After a time, they became partially paralyzed, which rendered her quite helpless.

When she came to me for treatment she was

unable to walk. I removed the metal jacket, and, by manipulation, strengthened the paralyzed muscles. By continuing this treatment three months she was able to walk perfectly, and the irritation had entirely disappeared from the spine.

In irritation, or weakness of the spine, it is not *bracing*, or *holding* strength, that we want, but lifting, or that the weight be taken off from the spine and the muscles left at liberty, whereby they can exercise themselves, and thus rouse their dormant powers ; then manipulation may be applied with every prospect of success.

The following cases may prove interesting. It gives me great pleasure to publish them :

DOUBLE SPINAL CURVATURE.

Miss G., a young lady, twenty-one years of age, crossed the ocean with her parents, who are wealthy, to consult European specialists as to the treatment necessary for her particular affliction ; namely, double spinal curvature.

She remained in Europe under the care of physicians about three years, but without good results. Returning to America, she spent five years more under physicians' care, but still the deformity existed.

Then she came to me for treatment. I removed the heavy iron support that had been placed upon the spine, and substituted a stiff whalebone corset,—as iron is injurious, because it tends to paralyze the muscles when coming in contact with them. Then, by manipulating the muscles of the spine, the contracted cords straigtened out, and the spinal column gradually resumed its original position. A three months' course of treatment succeeded in doing what years of medical attention had failed to accomplish.

TRIPLE CURVATURE.

Mrs. G., of Flushing, L. I., was among the most pitiful cases of triple curvature that I ever saw. The affliction had been of three or four years' duration.

It is supposed that this terrible distortion originated by using high pillows while sleeping, and by other causes of a similar nature. As to

her treatment, it had been the best, and everything any respectable authority could suggest had
been adopted. Laces, iron corsets, supports, etc.,
were used, but without success. When she came
to me she was encased in an iron corset of at
least twenty-five pounds weight, which her doctor
had instructed her to wear continually.

This I removed, and in its place used a stiff,
yielding corset of whalebone, which, as before
mentioned, permits an elasticity of movement,
very essential in curing diseases of the spine.

I never allow any metal to come in contact
with the body, when symptoms of paralysis or
contraction exist.

By removing the contraction from the cords,
and regulating the organs, within six months'
time she could walk perfectly straight.

CASE OF CONTRACTED LIMB.

Miss H., aged 13, was a beautiful and interesting girl; her skin very fair, and her flesh
plump and soft. She was perfect in form with
the exception of the lower limbs, one of which

was three and a half inches shorter than the other.

Desiring to correct this deformity, which dated from birth, she was placed under the care of an eminent physician when four years old, who, in order to lengthen the limb, attached an iron support of fifty pounds weight, bearing downwards. This was worn for years without producing the desired effect.

At length, when failing in health, I was called to attend her; I found the limb entirely paralyzed, possessing no feeling at all.

Her parents, having so much confidence in the physician, would not permit me to remove the iron support. After attending her a few months her health improved, their confidence in me increased, and I was permitted to remove the iron.

By manipulating and stretching the cords; not by heavy iron weights, but with my hands, within six months time I succeeded in lengthening the limb the desired three and a half inches.

Both limbs are now of the same length,

although the deformed limb does not possess the same power as the other, owing to the injurious effect of the iron band which the physician attached, pressing upon the muscles.

However, from present prospects, within a few more months' treatment, the deformity will then have been entirely removed.

CASE OF SUPPOSED DISLOCATION.

This case may prove interesting to those of my readers who imagine that when the " doctor " says so and so is the case, there remains no doubt with them but that his decision is strictly correct, and admitting of no doubt. Of course, the doctor expresses his opinion in good faith, and thinks he " knows all about it," but in many cases the doctors do not thoroughly examine the patient to find out where the trouble exists.

Though it is well known that my practice is confined strictly to the treatment of women and children, yet, when my attention was called to this case by one of my patients, and finally, when the mother so earnestly begged me to assist her boy, if possible, I consented to attend him.

The facts are these: her son, a lad of thirteen, while exercising on a horizontal bar, in a gymnasium, fell to the floor, a distance of six feet, and striking partially on his head, was removed to his home in an unconscious condition. A doctor was called to attend him who, after a superficial examination, pronounced the injury a " dislocation of the spine."

After remaining in a suffering condition for weeks and months, and experiencing no relief whatever, his vitality decreased, his strength became less and less, and the doctor, on being appealed to, said there was no help for him.

On my arrival, I found the tongue very dry and thickly coated with a white substance. This, the doctor said, came from the *stomach* (?) After thoroughly examining every cord and muscle, I found that the spine was not dislocated at all, but that the trouble was caused by the contraction, hardening, and diseased condition of several of the cords connected with the spine, and, as the muscles in the tongue are directly connected with the muscles of the spine, the thick coating formed on the tongue was due to the diseased condition of the cords and muscles, and did *not* emanate from the stomach, as the doctor said.

After removing by absorption, the diseased substances from the system, and by manipulating the contracted cords and muscles, the cords that before were dead and powerless gradually raised themselves and resumed their action.

After six weeks' treatment the young man was able to walk, and to-day is as well as he ever was.

Swelling of the Breast is not an unusual occurrence to women ; and, therefore, this case may be found interesting to some of my readers :

Some time ago a young lady, of one of our best New York families, while spending the summer at Long Branch, slightly injured one of her breasts, while in bathing. It is supposed that some substance was washed against her by the action of the waves. Soon afterward this injury compelled her to keep her bed. A physician was

called, who did all in his power to restore her to
health, but she gradually grew worse. At last
the physician told her she could not recover.
The sacrament was administered and nothing
remained, apparently, but to wait and watch her
death. On being advised by a friend, I was sent
for. I found her breast terribly swollen, and covered with some kind of salve, which the doctor had
prescribed. Removing this salve, and by gently
manipulating the breast and muscles of the entire
system, the swelling was gradually reduced, and
the breast grew smaller and smaller, day by day,
until at last they reached their normal condition,
and to-day she is well and enjoys excellent
health.

DISPLACEMENTS.

Only recently I had a patient under treatment who was troubled with displacement of the
womb. She had been under the care of physicians during the last four years, but without
obtaining relief.

When she came to me, a few months ago,
for treatment, I examined her thoroughly, and

found the direct cause of the displacement, due to the contraction of the cords extending from the point of the spine to the neck of the womb. The point of the spine had been injured, thereby causing the cords to contract ; and by the cords contracting, as a natural result, the womb was drawn from its proper position.   By manipulating these cords, they gradually became more elastic ; the contraction was removed, and the womb resumed its original position.

DISLOCATION OF THE SPINE.

Mrs. C., a very tall lady, residing in New York City, while entertaining some friends one evening, had occasion to visit the floor below, to give some instructions to the servants.

While passing hastily down the stairs, a misdirected step caused her to fall, when nearly down, resulting in a dislocation of the spine.

A physician was called to attend her, who neglected to thoroughly examine the spine, thereby failing to detect the existing dislocation ; and from the symptoms, described the'injury as merely *nervous prostration*, produced by the shock to her nervous system.

Different physicians were called, who blindly gave her drugs to cure some supposed ailment which did not exist.

After having been an invalid, and confined to her bed, for *eleven years*, I was called to attend her.

Examination revealed the fact of a deep cavity existing at the upper terminus of the spinal column, completely disconnecting the spine from the head—the result of a complicated dis-location. After four months' treatment, she re-covered sufficiently to go out, make calls, etc. ; another month's treatment completely restored her.

When the physicians who attended her, were informed of her complete restoration to health, the true cause of the disease, and the method of treatment employed, they expressed doubt as to the dislocation existing, and said that if it *had* existed, during all those years, such treatment would not remove it, in so short a time. When they had seen the patient they were convinced that the dislocation *had existed*, and also of their criminal negligence in not thoroughly examining the patient at first.

CASE OF INSANITY.

A lady, 26 years of age, whose family is well known in the best society of New York City, was so affected from some nervous ailment, as to be quite prostrated.

Her family physician was called in to attend her. To strengthen the nervous system he administered frequent doses of chloride; which, instead of having a beneficial effect, made the patient worse.

Another physician was called in—one of the first physicians in the city—who, in order to remove the effects of the chloride from the system, put on plasters.

The first plaster produced a soothing effect, after which he jokingly informed the patient that he "would use fifty more of the same kind." After using a few more, it so affected her brain as to cause her to refuse seeing any of her friends, and insist upon remaining in a darkened room all day ; her mind became affected and her speech became rambling and incoherent.

At this stage I was sent for. In order to assist manipulation, in strengthening the nervous system, I made a tea by boiling hops, and when cold placing in it a piece of iron, which I let remain until considerable rust had accumulated upon it ; this tea I poured into a sprinkling pot ; and removing her clothing, let the tea gently fall on the head and trickle down the body.

By repeating this operation daily, the desired effect was produced : the nervous system was strengthened and invigorated.

Then I removed the poison from the circulation by giving the patient rhubarb, and increased the supply of blood by the Milk Cure, which is administered as follows :

Let the patient deprive herself of the most unimportant meal each day, and take a glass or two of milk instead, for a week.

The second week, two meals should be dispensed with and milk used ; and the third week, milk should be used altogether.

It will be found that sufficient nourishment is obtained from milk alone, to support the constitution of a healthy person for any length of time, therefore the patient should have no fears of starvation from want of nourishment, when plenty of milk can be obtained.

The diet should be resumed in the same manner. Under my treatment the patient rapidly improved, and is now restored to perfect health.

RESULT OF EXPERIMENTS.

This case, which I have at present under treatment, is only a specimen of those which claim my attention, and which illustrate the evil results which sometimes follow the experiments of physicians.

The facts are these :

Miss C., of Connecticut, now a young lady of fourteen years, was rendered helpless at birth, by treatment herewith described, and has remained so ever since.

When born she possessed only the faintest spark of life, and some doubts were expressed as to her having any life. At length, when it was ascertained that life existed, the physicians, in order to fan this faint spark into a flame, immersed the new-born infant in *ice water*, and afterwards in *hot water*. This treatment resulted in a shrinkage of the spine, and contraction of the muscles and cords, making her completely helpless.

Nothing was done to correct this condition of affairs until she was a year old. Then she was treated by several well-known physicians of New York City, with but little or no success.

Six months ago her parents brought her to me for treatment. She could not stand erect, nor walk a step, nor talk, because of the muscles being so contracted. Now she can walk quite well without any support. She can talk, though imperfectly, and is rapidly improving. Within six months more she will be entirely cured.

I might go on to enumerate a host of cases in detail, but it is unnecessary, as many of the cases which have preceded, are in part of the same stamp, and much similarity exists in their treatment.

But I will say, that I firmly believe, millions in this country are now laboring under a set of chronic diseases, which are christened with names they do not deserve, but are merely a set of *effects* of one common cause, all requiring the same treatment, and that treatment is : support to the abdominal viscera and other organs by the strengthening of the muscles.

The experiments of doctors have been, and are, an important item of my practice ; therefore I should not speak unkindly, nor be too severe in the censuring of them, as without their assistance, my practice would never have risen to its present magnitude.

During the last ten years of my practice, I have successfully treated, by actual count (the records of which are in my possession,) *three hundred and eighty-five* patients suffering from some long-standing chronic disease, who had previously been under physicians' treatment, and pronounced incurable by them, and whose condition had only been aggravated by the experimental treatment received at their hands. Not a few have been those who were ruined by physicians' instruments, while undergoing an examination for some disease of the womb, or procreative organs.

Instruments should never be used in conducting an examination of these organs.

Many ladies in after life can trace the source of all their troubles, directly, to instruments employed by physicians in making an examination for some trifling ailment of these organs, in previous years.

The speculum, which is generally used by physicians in examining uterine derangements, has been the ruination of many young ladies.

Every physician should be so familiar with the location of the different organs, as to be able to detect any abnormal condition by the hands alone.

HINTS ON EVERY DAY ILLS.

Contraction of the rectum is one of the most common disorders to which ladies are subject, though least known. It is responsible for much of the pain, pressure, and weakness variously located in the spine, the ovaries, or at the base of the brain, which is so often complained of but unaccounted for. Sometimes it even occasions symptoms of insanity.

The cause of the contraction is not unfrequently due to an inactive or torpid liver. The main thing, then, is to restore a healthful action to that organ. Nothing will do this so quickly and safely, as plenty of out-door air and exercise. Walk regularly and perseveringly, and do not indulge in much carriage riding.

Skillful manipulation will also be very helpful. The contraction of the rectum will be much relieved by using an injection, made by steeping four large poppy heads and a tumblerful of bran in two quarts of water. Use this, cold, morning and evening.

Weakness of the Rectum is quite a common disorder, and is caused by the relaxation of the muscles employed in keeping it in position.

This weakness generally causes piles and similar disorders.

An excellent remedy for strengthening the rectum, and removing piles, is the following :

Pour a quart of water upon a pint of prepared tar, stir well, and when nearly cold, saturate a sponge and apply to the affected parts, at the same time pressing the organ upward ; use this every morning. Before retiring use sulphur soap instead, in the same manner. The tar used in making this application settles on the bottom, hence little of it is used, and a fresh quart of water can be poured upon it every morning for some time.

When the swelling is so aggravated as to prevent sitting down, use steamed hops instead, made by pouring three or four quarts of boiling water upon a tumblerful of hops.

The former treatment will sometimes aggravate the disease when first applied, but by continual applications, all the impurities will eventually be removed and a healthy reaction take place.

If the procreative and local organs are contracted, nothing will so readily remove the contraction as sitting for half an hour over steeped hops, after being strained, and deriving the benefit of the steam.

This treatment is also good for piles.

When the *womb*, or *bladder*, is relaxed, hop tea will be found very beneficial, used with alum and borax. The strength and quantity will depend very much upon the condition of the patient ; however, the average proportion may be estimated as follows : To one quart of hop tea add a tablespoonful of alum and a desertspoonful of borax ; shake well and use by saturating a sponge and applying to the affected organs, every evening before retiring.

The ovaries, or egg-bags, and the fallopian tubes, are subject to acute and chronic inflam-

mation ; but these affections are comparatively
less common than those of the womb.

The symptoms of inflammation in these parts
are very similar to those arising from inflammation of the womb, and the treatment is to be
conducted on the same general plan.

Pain, Oppression in Breathing, Palpitation,
and other *apparent* symptoms of heart disease,
often arise from irregularities of the spleen, which
produces an unequal circulation of the blood.

Manipulation should be applied in such a
manner as to assist the spleen (the office of which
is not unlike that of a sieve) in discharging the
blood which has been returned to it, after circulating through and nourishing the body.

This must be done, of course, by one who
understands the science of manipulation as well
as the theory of the circulation of the blood.

For Difficulty in Breathing, a feeling of dryness of the lungs, and other asthmatic symptoms,
mix a tablespoonful of anise-seed with two tablespoonfuls of honey, and a pint of cold milk ,and
take four tablespoonfuls daily.

It will remove the dryness from the throat, and give elasticity to the lungs.

The following is an excellent remedy for hemhorrages, weak lungs, inflamed throat, etc. :

Place a half pint of tar in two quarts of water, and boil down to about three pints ; when cold, strain off the water, letting the tar remain at the bottom, not using it ; add to the strained tar-water three pounds of loaf sugar, and boil down to about one quart ; then add half pint of gin or brandy.

Dose : A small wine-glassful three or four times a day, and less frequently as you improve.

For Sleeplessness and irritation of the nerves, take a cup of strong hop tea before retiring. It will tranquilize the nerves, and induce refreshing sleep, without being followed by any painful or depressing effects in the morning.

For quieting and strengthening the nerves and relaxing contractions of the stomach, I use, assisting manipulation, a preparation made from tincture of hops and camomile flowers, equal parts. A teaspoonful should be taken twice a day—in a half wine glass full of water—or often, according to the necessity of the case.

If much contraction and general debility exists, it may be taken several times a day with good results.

When *Neuralgic pain* in the head exists, temporary relief may be obtained by rubbing lemon juice well into the pores of the skin, both at the back of the head—where centre the nerves from the spine—and back of the ears. This nourishes and tranquilizes the nerves.

A radical cure can only be effected by enriching the blood, and generally building up the system. Spend more time in the open air, take more exercise, and thereby increase the appetite for nourishing food, of which eat as much as possible.

If you suffer with *Cold Feet*, do not use hot outward applications, or resort constantly to the register, but rub the feet briskly on the carpet or on a blanket, till the circulation is brought down to the extremities.

To *prevent* cold feet, wash them every night in cold water, with plenty of salt in it.

Tumors.—The most common in practice are:

the Blood Tumor, Muscular Tumor, Dropsical Tumor, and Fibrous Tumor.

I do not consider tumors dangerous, or even of a serious nature, as proper treatment will very readily remove them.

Blood tumors are generally produced by irregularity of the monthly courses, either by occurring too early or too late.

The blood not being properly discharged, clots and hardens in the ovaries, or left side below the spleen, and the tumor is formed.

An injection made from hop tea, with lemon juice added, will readily remove them.

Muscular tumors may appear at any part of the muscular system, where the muscles are disposed to contract. This is often caused by excessive stretching of the muscles. I have removed many muscular tumors that were caused by ladies carelessly crossing their lower limbs. The predisposition is often due to slight causes. Manipulation will readily remove them.

Dropsical tumors are generally concealed in the ovaries and womb. Excessive medical treatment will produce them.

Especially are those liable to this species of tumor, who use quinine ; as this tends to change the blood to water, and the excessive supply of water in these parts will produce a tumor.

The treatment is the same as that of the blood tumor.

Fibrous tumors are concealed in different parts of the abdomen and ovaries, and can easily be removed by manipulation, which has the effect of absorbing the tumor.

No operation is necessary, as the above treatment will invariably remove them.

Cancers are generally produced by a pressure on some fleshy part. A pressure on any portion of our body prevents the small fibres in the blood (which is the most important element of its composition) from passing through the system. When these collect together, because of the pressure, the cancer is formed. As long as these fibres can be separated they will not grow, but when permitted to collect, they grow together, day by day ; and when hardened, and the cancer has grown to any size, nothing but an operation will remove it.

If the operator is careful to remove all the fibres which have grown together, the cure will be permanent.

Scrofulous Cancer can never be cured, for the reason that the entire system is filled with these poisonous scrofulous fibres.

An operation would be a useless affliction to the patient, for when one is removed, another appears. ·

Sulphur baths will be found most beneficial, in connection with inhaling the steam of sulphur.

www.ingramcontent.com/pod-product-compliance
Lightning Source LLC
Chambersburg PA
CBHW021217270326
41929CB00010B/1168